ANGER MANAGEMENT FOR TEENAGERS

PRACTICAL STRATEGIES FOR PARENTS, EDUCATORS, AND TEENS TO BRIDGE THE COMMUNICATION GAP, CULTIVATE TRUST, AND HARMONIZE EMOTIONS

SASHA WOODLEY

CONTENTS

Introduction   7

1. UNDERSTANDING ANGER IN ADULTS AND
   TEENS   17
   Defining Adolescence   17
   What Is Anger?   19
   The Mechanics of Anger   19
   Anger as a Secondary Emotion   21
   Myths About Anger   23
   Expressions of Anger   24
   When Does Anger Become a Problem?   25
   Brain Structure 101   26
   The Teen Brain and Behavior   28
   Anger and the Teen Brain   28
   Dealing With Negative Emotions   32
   Will I Ever Feel Better?   33
   Positive Actions for Teens   33

2. TRIGGERED!   35
   Understanding Anger's Triggers   36
   Triggers for Teenage Anger   38
   Teen Stress and Anxiety   48
   When Anger Becomes Dangerous   53
   Positive Actions Teens Can Take   55

3. GETTING TO KNOW AND LOVE YOURSELF   59
   Understanding Teen Moodiness   60
   Dealing With Stress and Anxiety as a Teenager   63
   Overcoming Social Anxiety   68
   Successfully Navigating Challenges as a Teenager   71
   Learning to Love Yourself   72
   Becoming Self-Aware   74
   Learning to Say "No"   77
   Eating for Optimism and Positivity   78

Success Stories   83
Positive Actions Teens Can Take   84

4. DEFUSING THE BOMB   89
How Do We Know We Are Triggered?   90
What to Do When You Are Triggered   91
Controlling Your Thoughts   91
Changing Your Beliefs   93
Letting Things Go   94
The Problem of Toxic Positivity   94
Resolving Adolescent Conflicts and Triggers   95
Success Stories   104
Positive Actions Teens Can Take   106

5. EMOTIONAL CATCH AND RELEASE   107
Suppressing Anger   108
Anger and Other Emotions   109
Releasing Strong Emotions Safely   114
Three-Step NPR Action   120
It Stops With You   123

6. JEDI MIND TRICKS   125
Success Stories: Finding Your Zen   126
Mindfulness for Anger Management   127
Developing Mindfulness   130
Success Story: Chores and Privileges   133

7. ADULTING TEENAGERS   135
Parents Versus Teens—Anger Triggers From a
Parent's Perspective   137
Authoritative Parenting: The Best Parenting Style   141
Creating Win-Win Situations   143
Tips for Communicating With Teens   145
Appreciating Who Teens Are   147
Developing Problem-Solving Skills in Teens   148

8. CASE STUDIES—SUCCESS STORIES   151
Life-Changing Teen Anger   151
Building a Stronger Teen-Parent Relationship   153
Building a Relationship With a Rebellious,
Troubled Teen   154

Conclusion   157

References   161

INTRODUCTION

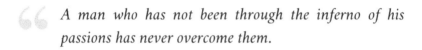 *A man who has not been through the inferno of his passions has never overcome them.*

— CARL JUNG

Commenting on a YouTube video about adolescence, Abby says, "I'm eighteen, and sometimes I want to scream at my older family members and get them to remember their adolescence. Because I know they had these same feelings—feeling out of control, lost, having no faith in themselves" (Abby, 2022).

A 13-year-old boy tells an online psychologist that everything is making him mad. He is getting angry over stupid things. If someone shouts at him, he yells back louder. But there could be a reason for his anger. He goes on to explain that other kids at school are kicking him, pushing him, and throwing him against school lockers. He is being bullied. He doesn't know what to do, so he resorts to anger.

On the same site, a father expresses concern about his 11-year-old son, who is good at sports but became aggressive after being bullied at school (DeFoore, n.d.). His son is expressing his anger inappropriately at sports games and is being excluded from teams. The father worries that his son's behavior will make him an isolated, lonely teen.

Anger is often considered a negative emotion, but seeing it in a more positive light is essential. It generates a surge of energy, and if we learn to harness it, we can use it to generate positivity. When we understand our emotions, we can rise above them and live life to the fullest.

TEENAGE YEARS ARE DIFFICULT

Many teens feel their parents—and other adults—don't understand them. They think their parents don't accept or adhere to the boundaries they might set with their elders. Parents also wonder why they can't get along with their teens. While adolescents can be moody, this is not always caused by hormonal changes. Depression and anxiety are increasing among young adults. One of my friend's teenagers says nearly all his friends constantly talk about how anxious they feel.

Several things trigger teen anxiety:

- There is tremendous pressure to succeed due to standardized testing and the practice of rewarding achievement. In 2016, 41% of first-year college students said they felt overwhelmed compared to 28% in 2000 and 18% in 1985 (McCarthy, 2019).
- The world we live in makes young people feel frightened and unsafe. Occurrences of mass shootings, school shootings, and terrorist attacks have mushroomed. There are lockdowns and drills at places of learning.
- Today's adolescents constantly interact on social media. Their self-esteem and worldview may be influenced by what others do, making them feel inadequate.
- Some children always felt a little anxious, with everyday experiences enough to set them off. This worsens during puberty.

If high anxiety remains unaddressed, it might engender depression, substance abuse, and even suicide. One teen expressed her opinion on social media that Gen Z and millennials have some of the highest rates of depression, anxiety, and suicide in our society. Another added that her family doesn't know how to respond when she feels depressed or anxious, so she gravitates toward her friends.

Adolescence is when young people come to grips with the real world. While this can be exciting, it can also be daunting, leaving many teens at a loss. Some perceive that adulthood might not be quite as glamorous as they anticipated. Teenagers are sometimes expected to shoulder some of their parents' responsibilities.

Teens are very aware of their insecurities and vulnerabilities and often discuss them with their peers. The need to conform is intense and often puts teens in challenging positions. While they are mature enough to understand the reasons for their actions, they might make poor decisions because they lack life experience. All this adds to their stress and anxiety.

WHY ARE TEENS SO ANGRY?

Teenagers experience numerous physical and emotional changes as they move toward adulthood. While anger is a normal human emotion, it can be devastating if it is inappropriately expressed. Some teens lose friends due to their constant angry outbursts. Beneath the anger, low self-esteem, anxiety, depression, childhood abuse, and old grudges may lurk. Many teens with anger issues feel they cannot be themselves as they must live up to their parents' expectations.

They may feel pressured to perform well at school to attend colleges their parents have selected. Some might need to care for the adults in their lives who may be incapable due to bereavement, substance abuse, or being estranged from the family and friends who could support them.

While such teens may hide their anger, pain, or resentment beneath a cloak of apparent willingness and cheerfulness, it's just a veneer. Beneath it, they are constantly simmering. One day, the volcano may erupt. At least some teens believe their anger was inherited because one or both of their parents are angry adults.

All this is very confusing for teens caught in anger's relentless grip. Many feel helpless and alone. Their outbursts make them feel guilty and ashamed. Some don't know why they are so angry, while others have buried painful childhood memories of abuse, absent parents, grief, and other difficult experiences.

In addition, many teens have ineffective adult role models and, therefore, do not know—or have never been taught—how to regulate their emotions. They don't know what anger is, what it means, or how to manage it. It doesn't help that anger is often glamorized in the media.

Young adults frequently don't know how to set boundaries—or what to do when someone transgresses a boundary they've developed. They can't let go of past wrongs and their anger burns. They find it hard to calm down after outbursts, and the aftermath may linger for days.

Angry teens could lose out on opportunities because of their aggressive behavior. People might avoid them, and they may end up becoming lonely and isolated.

WHAT PARENTS CAN DO

Parents need to do more with and for their teenagers as these are often stressful years. It's a time of tremendous change—social changes reflected in their relationships and friendships and physical changes that make them sexually aware and appearance-conscious. Today's teens face high academic demands and expectations, peer pressure, and parental rules like curfews and study time. The resultant anxiety and stress often manifest as resentment and anger, much of it directed toward parents.

When I look back on my own teenage years, I believe we do our teens a disservice by attributing their grievances and responses to the world around them. Teenagers should be a valuable litmus test for parents and society as they react to real things. We sometimes need to take a deeper look at what's really going on.

Parents should not define their children by their negative behaviors—door slamming, eyes rolling, swearing, cheekiness, etc. Don't send mixed messages. For example, don't encourage teens to talk about contentious subjects and, when they do, tell them they're not supposed to know about such things because they are just children.

Teen anger has its reasons, but so does parental frustration; the issues can be resolved. If you opt for anger management sessions, it is essential to realize that a certain amount of excess emotion with no apparent basis will emerge. Focus on solving the problems rather than your feelings to build a better relationship.

Many studies show a teen's anger issues might be rooted in childhood. How strong was the bond between parent and child? How are the parents dealing with the changes in their child? The transition from childhood to adulthood requires a certain amount of autonomy if children are going to become mature, responsible adults.

Being a teenager is not merely a life phase. This is when we build the skills and knowledge needed for transitioning into adulthood. If teen anger isn't handled correctly, teens will take these potentially destructive emotions into the next phase of their lives.

If parents want to treat teenagers as equals as adults, trust them and allow them to explore and make mistakes. If parents are prepared to be their safety net if things go wrong, their teens will be happier. That is one of the reasons I love my parents so much. They let me make my own decisions and helped me cope with the consequences while growing into adulthood. This enabled me to learn from experience without being knocked over by the full impact of a poor choice.

HOW THIS BOOK CAN HELP YOU

One of the teenagers' most common complaints is that nobody understands them, while most parents struggle to relate to their teenage children. This book will delve into that conflict, providing tips on how to improve these all-important relationships.

Some teens wonder why they are so moody and if they'll feel like this forever. They wonder if it's because of technology, social media, or their hormones. I will answer this question in this book.

I am deeply invested in the well-being of our youth, regularly participating in seminars and podcasts hosted by family counselors and mental health therapists. My certification in Youth Mental Health First Aid (YMHFA) further reflects this commitment. Alarmingly, the teenage mental health crisis in the United States appears to be escalating. The National Alliance on Mental Illness in Texas reports a 31% increase in emergency room visits related to mental health since February 2022. Moreover, students between the ages of 6 and 17 with mental, emotional, or behavioral disturbances are three times more likely to repeat a grade (Anger Issues in Teen Girls, n.d.).

Beyond these alarming statistics, specific events in my community have underscored the gravity of this issue. Not long ago, and within just 24 hours, two teenage girls attending a local university committed suicide (Chuck, 2023). One of the students messaged a friend to say she was considering taking her own life. Her body was later found near a local lake. In the other instance, there is little information beyond the fact that the teen had spoken to friends shortly before her suicide. The university chancellor said the incidents were heartbreaking. In 2018, a promising college-bound student who lived close to one of my friends was sentenced to 12 years in prison for suffocating his mother in their garage (Charles & Lamb, 2018). News reports alleged that the mother had verbally and physically abused her son for years, and he finally snapped, choking her to death. A lawyer interviewed by a local paper suggested that the student had been keeping his anger bottled up for a long time.

These heart-wrenching stories, coupled with the dire statistics, accentuate the urgency of the situation. I've engaged with our youth for over a decade with this understanding and urgency. For the past decade, I've mentored numerous high school interns and am also the parent of a 13-year-old daughter. It's a privilege to share the wisdom and insights I've gained from interacting with and raising young individuals. I sincerely wish for this book to serve as a beacon, guiding parents and teens toward nurturing relationships amidst the ever-present challenges that could distance us from one another.

This book offers straightforward anger management and self-regulation strategies that teenagers, parents, and educators can easily understand and implement. It also guides parents in fostering positive, fulfilling relationships with their adolescent children.

"Remember that our kids are our future. We need to be there for them and show them the way" (Ambar, 2022).

1

UNDERSTANDING ANGER IN ADULTS AND TEENS

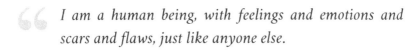

I am a human being, with feelings and emotions and scars and flaws, just like anyone else.

— JOSH GORDON

There are several reasons why teenagers become angry. Although teens experience and express anger differently from adults because their brains are still developing, it is an emotion like any other, such as happiness or surprise. It's critical to recognize that anger is a secondary emotion and establish what underpins this response.

DEFINING ADOLESCENCE

Adolescence is a time of transition when children become adults, starting with puberty. The word comes from a Latin verb meaning "to mature." Even though teenagers are usually considered adolescents, this process may start earlier or continue into one's 20s. Therefore, The World Health Organization defines adolescents as those aged 10–19 (Wikipedia Contributors, 2019).

History of Adolescence

There was only sometimes a transition period between childhood and adulthood. Between the fifth and 16th centuries, when girls reached 14, they were considered legal adults. For example, they could sign contracts, get married, or claim inheritances. However, men were only regarded as legal adults when they were 21. In later centuries, children as young as nine were sent into service, working in a wealthy person's household or learning a trade (Carlson et al., n.d.). By the end of adolescence, most people were already working in their lifetime trades or jobs.

Psychologist G. Stanley Hall coined the term "adolescence" in 1904 to refer to young people aged between 14 and 24. By the end of that decade, children were legally obliged to remain in school until they were 14 years old. In the early 1940s, the term "teenager" came into general use (Carlson et al., n.d.).

The word ultimately became a marketing gimmick. After World War II, the role of young people in society changed. They became a separate group with their own needs, desires, and values. In the 1950s, commercial companies realized they could tap into this potentially lucrative market from which trendsetters, fashionistas, and influencers would emerge (Fisher, 2022). What better way to market products than to exploit the needs, desires, and concerns of vulnerable young people who want to conform with one another?

Some cultures have rites of passage where children are recognized as adults. These experiences help bridge the gap between childhood and adulthood, acknowledging these young adults' contribution to a particular society.

WHAT IS ANGER?

Understanding the foundations of anger and how to deal with it benefits everyone, not only teenagers. According to the American Psychological Association, anger is an emotion characterized by antagonism toward someone or something you feel has deliberately done you wrong (n.d.). The association says that about 25% of anger incidents involve vengeful thoughts to "get even" or "put them in their place" (2021).

For example, anger often results when someone feels threatened, disrespected, or betrayed. Anger triggers the body's fight-or-flight response. It is a normal, healthy emotion, not a mental illness.

THE MECHANICS OF ANGER

Anger is one of five basic emotions—anger, fear, sadness, disgust, and enjoyment—that are found in most human cultures (*Basic Emotions*, n.d.). These emotions appear in early childhood and are believed to be a substitute for the survival instincts found in most living creatures. Emotions such as anger and fear alert us to dangerous, potentially harmful situations. Our senses constantly monitor the surrounding environment for potential threats. When one is detected, a message is sent to the amygdala in the brain, associated with emotions like fear, anxiety, and anger. This prepares the body for a fight-or-flight response. The process is entirely unconscious, and that is how anger is created biologically.

After this, another message is transmitted to the cerebral cortex —the part of the brain that processes our thoughts. We evaluate the nature of the threat and choose what to do. This is the reaction part of anger. The fight-or-flight response is triggered if we decide an aggressive or hostile reaction is required.

Our bodies react to threatening situations by releasing hormones like adrenaline and cortisol. Cortisol is manufactured and released by the adrenal cortex, the outermost section of the adrenal glands located above the kidneys. Hormones like adrenaline (or epinephrine) are catecholamines produced by the adrenal medulla in the brain and some nerve fibers. Adrenaline rapidly increases the heart rate and respiration, and it causes other subtle changes in the body as well. Cortisol is released more slowly, over hours or days. The hormone norepinephrine signals its release to prepare the body for long-term stress. Cortisol inhibits growth and reproduction and changes the body's metabolism to enable quick action or preparation for future famine by raising blood sugar levels and increasing fat storage.

These biological responses put us on alert and speed up our reactions. They limit blood flow to the torso and send more to the arms and legs, enabling us to run from an enemy or other threat. Our blood pressure and body temperature will also rise.

This is when anger erupts, sometimes volcanically. Our brain chemistry reflects our emotions. Cortisol decreases when we feel joyful—the brain releases serotonin in response to our positive emotions. We feel calm, comfortable, and focused when serotonin levels are optimal.

ANGER AS A SECONDARY EMOTION

Often referred to as a secondary emotion, anger is complex, frequently spurred by other feelings, with fear, sadness, or disgust lurking beneath the fury, like some psychological Loch Ness monster. We nearly always feel something else before we get angry. We perceive the entire emotion as anger if these feelings are intense enough. A good example is when someone cuts us off while driving in heavy traffic. Most of us immediately feel angry. Almost no one recognizes that in that millisecond before we sounded the horn or took evasive action, we felt a spurt of fear that our physical safety could be jeopardized by a vehicle accident. In reality, anger is like an iceberg (see Figure 1) in that only some emotions are apparent. The vast majority are hidden below the waterline, where they are not immediately evident to others or ourselves.

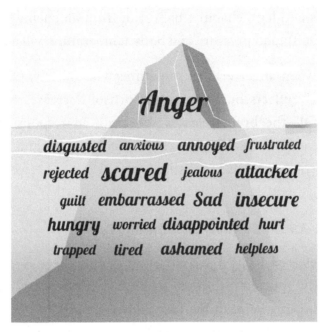

Figure 1

If you are confident about who you are and know your value, you do not need to fear changes in your circumstances. If others say something offensive, you won't take it personally. You won't be concerned with what others think when your conscience is clear. You won't get jealous if you know you have good skills and are doing your best.

Anger might also result from our interpretation of and reactions to situations. There are several reasons why we interpret a particular situation; finding out how and why can help us better manage our emotions.

Anger frequently masks those other feelings to protect us from them, cloaking our vulnerability. Teens may hide feelings like sadness beneath anger because expressing anger is much more comfortable. Parents need to show them how to deal with their emotions constructively.

MYTHS ABOUT ANGER

Because it is such a strong emotion, anger has collected its fair share of myths over time. Before continuing, it's worth taking a look at them. You may conform to some of these beliefs, which makes managing this powerful emotion and seeing it in perspective more challenging.

Anger Is Negative

Anger is not necessarily a bad thing. All emotions are essential —we need to have feelings. For instance, positive things like social change happen because someone gets angry. It can also motivate you to do better. Being aggressive when angry isn't a positive expression of your feelings.

Venting Your Anger Releases It

Anger expresses itself physically. Angry people might get sweaty, breathless, or red-faced. They might imagine that screaming, shouting, and punching or throwing things will make them feel better. It won't. Expressing anger physically actually inflames it, creating a vicious circle.

Ignoring Your Anger Will Kill It

Ignoring your anger doesn't make it disappear. Those who ignore their anger and frustration or allow others to mistreat them can drive themselves ill. Many medical conditions, from hypertension to depression, result from suppressing and ignoring angry feelings.

Anger Is Inherited

Anger is an emotion and a character trait, so it can't be inherited. People who grow up seeing people destructively react when angry might do the same because of their background. This doesn't mean they are hardwired for anger.

Other People Can Make You Angry

Many people blame their feelings on others when they are triggered. Their interpretation of a situation—which often happens subconsciously—makes them react angrily.

EXPRESSIONS OF ANGER

- Anger can be expressed assertively when the angry person gets their point across without resorting to threats.
- Some people may become very aggressive when angry and act violently toward others, animals, or objects.

- Passive anger is just another term for suppressing anger.

WHEN DOES ANGER BECOME A PROBLEM?

Anger is a fierce emotion that can rapidly escalate into hostility, aggression, and even violence. This is when anger becomes a problem, as others might be harmed. Unexpressed or suppressed anger can also be an issue.

Many people don't realize that anger does not have to be expressed by a volcanic eruption but can be a simple statement of fact (Woodley, 2023). It's enough to make a factual statement that a specific action or behavior has made one angry without yelling, slamming doors, or throwing things.

Many schools traditionally haven't emphasized teaching children and teens about managing their emotions in the same formalized way they teach subjects like math or history. Youngsters learn these skills at home, with their parents and caregivers as teachers and role models. Angry parents are more inclined to raise angry offspring, whereas calmer parents will likely raise more emotionally balanced young adults.

According to research conducted at McLean Hospital, innocuous angry outbursts can harm children's developing brains (Dougherty, n.d.). Even verbal abuse can scar the brain— with the fallout lasting well into adulthood. The effects are similar to witnessing acts of domestic violence and sexual abuse. Children may become physically ill, while adolescents could develop anxiety, depression, anger, and hostility and are more likely to abuse drugs or alcohol. Unbridled anger can be traumatic to watch. Children's brains diminish the experience, causing specific sensory pathways to function less effectively. While psychiatry focuses on issues like anxiety and depression, the real problem is the anger they cloak—and the negative experiences or perceptions beneath.

BRAIN STRUCTURE 101

Before we continue, it's crucial to understand how the brain develops during adolescence.

Human brains are the largest among all living beings, with the cerebral cortex being the most significant part of this organ. The brain regulates and controls all the body's functions, interprets information from the outside world via the senses, and contains the mind and soul. It has three parts—the cerebrum, the cerebellum, and the brainstem. The brain is part of the central nervous system, which includes the spinal cord.

Let's focus on the prefrontal cortex (see Figure 2) and the limbic system. As the name suggests, the former is located in the front of the brain's frontal lobe. The limbic system is hidden deep inside the brain, beneath the cerebral cortex and above the brainstem. This part of the brain includes the hippocampus and amygdala, structures that keep your body in a stable state or homeostasis (see Figure 2). They do this by directly influencing your autonomic nervous system and controlling your hormones.

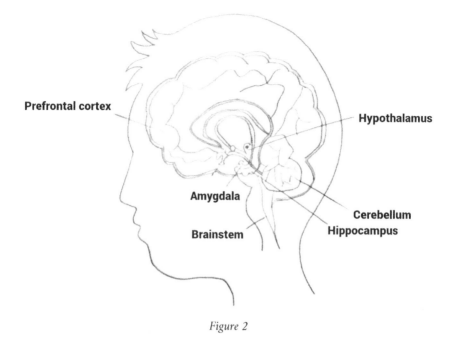

Figure 2

The prefrontal cortex determines personality, goals, and values, ensuring the development of healthy relationships. It controls reasoning, conferring the ability to make decisions and judgments, solve problems, understand the physical world, and develop self-control and perseverance. It is also the seat of creativity. The limbic system regulates behavioral and emotional responses.

The brain consists of two types of cells: nerve cells (neurons) and glial cells. The latter defines the structure of the brain. Neurons are messengers that use chemical and electrical signals to send information to the central nervous system and the rest of the body. Each neuron has a long cable called an axon that allows nerve cells to send electrical and chemical signals to other nerves, glands, and muscle cells. Neurons have spikes called dendrites that pick up messages from other nerve cells (see Figure 3).

THE TEEN BRAIN AND BEHAVIOR

"I vividly remember my teenage years. My friends and I always acted as though we were intoxicated or weird from staying up all night or something, and our parents were very embarrassing, no matter what they did" (Peter, 2022).

Parents might become concerned when they see their teens doing peculiar things, but this means that their brains are developing correctly. For example, teens might suddenly get embarrassed about being seen with their parents and could become frustrated with them. Although this is hurtful, their brains create a healthy emotional distance that will make it easier for them to transition to adulthood, become independent, and leave the family home. This might also make teens say they hate their parents, which might be painful to hear but is untrue.

ANGER AND THE TEEN BRAIN

The process of anger is different in teenagers, whose brains are still maturing. The limbic system is not fully developed and disconnected from the brain's rational parts. These connections form later in life. In addition, the two systems mature at different rates.

Like a mental conspiracy theorist, the amygdala fires up, planting false news in teenagers' minds and making them believe that everyone is against them. Adding fuel to the fire, the hypothalamus (see Figure 2) goes into overdrive, loading the body with sex hormones, particularly testosterone, which increases hostility. The amygdala becomes even more frantic in making teens believe its conspiracies, blowing everything out of proportion. The unchecked rampaging of the limbic brain makes teens feel like caged lions, well out of their comfort zones in a strange environment. A teen might even see a benign "hello" as a battle cry. If the basketball coach is not clearly smiling, an adolescent might erroneously conclude that the coach hates him.

The excess hormones create mood swings, which can be very perplexing for teenagers, who can't understand why they feel vaguely bipolar much of the time. Girls may burst into tears for no apparent reason, for example.

There are ways of controlling the runaway limbic system to strengthen the communication between it and the prefrontal cortex. Hand model of the brain (Siegel, 2017) is a handy tool that visualizes how our brain works and helps us better understand our emotions. I will talk about how to apply it in Chapter 5. The proper guidance from parents, education, and opportunities also play a role.

Once a person reaches their early 20s, the more rational part of the brain (the prefrontal cortex) starts controlling the limbic system, preventing the latter from overreacting. The prefrontal cortex fully develops by age 25 (Arain et al., 2013).

Other changes in the teenage brain also affect behavior. While children's brains are focused on increasing neurons and the connections between them, making the brain more efficient, the opposite happens in puberty. The brain culls neurons and their connections in a process known as pruning (Dalai Lama Center for Peace and Education, 2014).

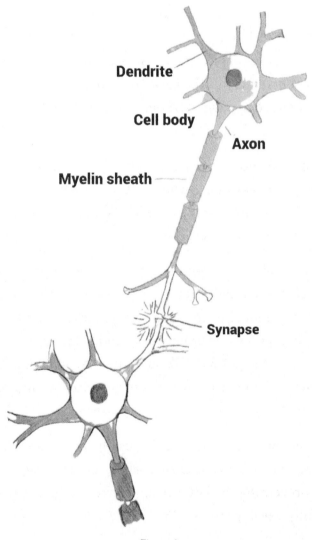

Figure 3

The myelin sheath begins forming during adolescence (see Figure 3). It is a soft material covering the axon in a protective layer of protein and fatty substances (lipids). The Myelin sheath works similarly to the insulation on an electrical cord, facilitating the quick, efficient movement of electrical impulses between nerve cells and maintaining their strength. The communication between such circuits is 3,000 times faster than circuits without myelin (Dalai Lama Center for Peace and Education, 2014), which helps streamline brain functioning. These brain changes help teens cope with unfamiliar, uncomfortable, and even unsafe environments, paving the way to becoming independent adults.

When neurons communicate, they release dopamine, a chemical messenger (neurotransmitter), and a hormone. Dopamine is often associated with pleasure but also motivates certain behaviors, like learning and working behaviors, and long-term memory. For example, we get a dopamine spike if we find something interesting. This makes it easier to remember things we find fascinating.

The dopamine release in teen brains encourages them to try new things and promotes hyper-rational thinking biased toward risky behaviors. Because the brain and nervous system are remodeled during adolescence, teens feel more emotional, often becoming angry quickly and frequently. Low dopamine levels in the brain may also contribute to attention deficit disorders such as ADD.

Knowing what happens in teen brains helps us understand why many teens engage in risky behaviors. While they usually are physically fit and have robust immune systems, death rates may increase by as much as 200–300% after childhood ends (AsapSCIENCE, 2016). Typical causes of death include road accidents, homicide, and suicide. Mental illnesses like anxiety, depression, and eating disorders often begin during adolescence.

DEALING WITH NEGATIVE EMOTIONS

People generally want to avoid uncomfortable or painful emotions, hoping they will disappear. Distractions like engaging in a frenetic activity or using alcohol or drugs worsen them. Once the distraction is over, the feelings return in full force. It's better to feel the emotions and work through them.

Anger occurs for a reason. By suppressing it, the pain or feelings underlying it (remember, anger is a secondary emotion) are ignored, which might cause depression. Avoiding the anger and painful emotions could reduce empathy. A 2011 study established that more sociable individuals are less likely to get angry or suppress anger (Golden, 2020).

It takes a surprising amount of effort and energy to suppress anger. Such people may be less present, affecting all their relationships and work performance. The problem often starts when children are prevented from expressing their feelings or ridiculed when they do. The emotions gradually build up and explode, dismaying and confusing those around them.

WILL I EVER FEEL BETTER?

If you are a teen—or the parent of one—struggling with anger, I can reassure you that you will, but only if you work with your emotions. Using the tips and tools in this book will help you feel better over time. Consider it as a building block. The more blocks there are, the stronger you will ultimately be.

Find an outlet for your anger so you don't lash out randomly. Doing something physical is generally very helpful. Go for a walk or participate in a sport (for me, it is running and boxing). Some individuals might prefer to write (keeping an emotional journal can be helpful—I'll explain how to do that in Chapter 3), draw, do yoga, or meditate. Find an activity that works for you.

POSITIVE ACTIONS FOR TEENS

The next time you get angry, analyze what happened when you have calmed down.

- Identify the thoughts you had before you got angry.
- What was your physical state? Were you tired, hungry, or thirsty at the time?
- What made you feel angry?
- What emotions did you feel, and how intense were they? Did you sense anything in your body? If so, where?
- Look at your thoughts. What disturbed you? Were there any images, thoughts, or memories that came to you?

What are you responding to, and what is the worst thing that could happen?

- Look at the facts. Do they support your thoughts or not? Were these thoughts based on reality or not?
- Reason about the situation. Consider what others might do when faced with it. What's the bigger picture? Could you perceive the situation differently? What advice would you give someone in this situation?
- Is your reaction out of proportion with what happened? How important is this for you?
- Lastly, consider how you are now feeling. Are you calmer and more relaxed, or are you still outraged?
- If you experience this again, what would you do? Is there a more effective way to deal with this? What would the consequences of your actions be?

It can be helpful to write this down so you can clarify your thoughts and feelings. This will enable you to understand yourself better and how you relate to others.

2

TRIGGERED!

> *If we become aware of what's happening before we act, behavior becomes a function of choice rather than a result of an impulse or trigger. You begin to control your world more than the outside world controlling you.*
>
> — MARSHALL GOLDSMITH

What makes us angry? Teens are likely to get angry when their parents, teachers, or other authority figures try to control the things they do. When friends let them down, peers gossip about them, or they get bullied on social media, they'll probably get mad. If there's a lot of conflict in a family, such people get angry more quickly than others. If someone has passed away, grief could manifest as anger.

Anger has numerous triggers—teens react to them the same way as adults do. However, adolescents get angry more often because their brains are developing. They're trying to assert themselves, build their identities, and discover what makes them unique. These things can add to teens' stressors, compounding their potential for fueling anger and aggression.

UNDERSTANDING ANGER'S TRIGGERS

There are two types of triggers—visible and invisible triggers.

- **Visible triggers** are situations or events that make us feel threatened, frustrated, powerless, or disrespected. For example, I might respond angrily when my friends laugh at me, I break my sunglasses, or I cannot find my favorite toothbrush. Everyone interprets situations differently, so something that makes one person feel angry might not make another person angry at all. How people react to a situation depends on their childhood experiences, their past, and their current circumstances.
- This is where **invisible triggers** come in. These originate from unresolved painful events in the past. For example, anger may be triggered by hurtful childhood memories that have been suppressed. As a teen, your parents' anger might have been out of control, but you were not allowed to complain or express your feelings because you were a child. A good example is the children of abusive parents, who may suffer from low self-esteem and feel insecure. These feelings might drive teens to lash out in anger or rage. If you consider the iceberg analogy, these would be the below-the-waterline feelings. Studies show that people

who get angry quickly sometimes did not receive enough love and care during infancy.

According to a friend with over 25 years of experience in psychotherapy, most of her clients' emotional problems are rooted in childhood events or trauma that have never been resolved (Woodley, 2023). Our bodies also react when something is wrong—we may suffer from unexplained aches and pains and generally have poor health.

Becoming angry for no apparent reason may indicate someone is dealing with an invisible trigger. In Chapter 4, we will discuss how to deal with these triggers.

A visible trigger could also stimulate an invisible one, which is why people sometimes get angry at seemingly trivial things. If someone's hidden triggers are unresolved, tiny and insignificant things tend to spark their anger.

There are a few reasons why people might explode without warning:

- Those who get angry quickly are often insecure and have low self-esteem. Their fear drives them to lash out. This happens when people haven't developed mechanisms to cope in more positive ways.
- Irritability can be a sign of stress or unhappiness. When people feel significantly stressed, small things push them over the edge, and they lash out. It's easier for people to resort to anger than to look more deeply into their feelings.

- Those who have a short fuse may find it difficult to compromise.
- Intolerant people often anger easily. They realize too late that everything is solvable, regardless of the situation. Based on my observations, people who overthink, calculate, and look for faults are most likely to be angered easily.
- Anger manifests when we feel we have lost control. Most often, what people feel when they blow off steam is not anger but a much more destructive emotion —rage.

TRIGGERS FOR TEENAGE ANGER

Today's teens are angry for several reasons. They struggle with social problems in much the same way as adults do. However, teens have trouble processing that information because their brains still develop while their bodies mature. Sometimes, the latter outstrips the former. This situation may be exacerbated by stress and anxiety. Let's unpack some of the reasons why today's teens seem to be angrier than previous generations.

Effects of the COVID-19 Pandemic

The COVID-19 pandemic had a particularly negative impact on teenagers. By March 2020, around 91% of schools worldwide were closed, and many remained through a large part of 2021 (Bose, 2023). The confinement, restrictions on activities and educational disruption exacerbated adolescents' uncertainties. Some teens were exposed to domestic and emotional abuse. For students who were homeschooled or attended virtual school, connecting with teachers and peers proved challenging. In fact, almost 70% found it harder to complete assignments (Leamey, 2022).

All this has impacted teens' mental health. Depression and anxiety in children and teens surged by around 32% during the pandemic (Bose, 2023). With no face-to-face opportunities to interact with peers, young people internalized their problems more than before. There was a 51% increase in emergency room visits for adolescent girls who had attempted suicide (Leamey, 2022). Students who felt more connected, even virtually, fared better than those who didn't.

Studies have established that adolescent brains aged prematurely during the pandemic. The brains of teens who had experienced ten months of lockdown were found to have aged by around three years, equivalent to children who are neglected, subjected to violence, and come from dysfunctional families (*Teen Brains*, n.d.).

Prejudice and Labeling

Much teen anger stems from modern society's negative perceptions of adolescents, resulting in widespread prejudice. One teen complained on social media that her bags are checked every time she goes shopping. Often, the security personnel tell her they're checking that she has only been shopping and not stealing. She says people are rude, staring at her, and making assumptions about her that are not necessarily true. Another recounts an experience where a strange man told her she should be partying, wearing heels, and having boyfriends.

Teens don't like being labeled and dislike it when they are put into a one-size-fits-all box. They get upset when their emotions are dismissed as adolescent angst. What they are going through is real, painful, and confusing. It can be hurtful when they are told that their experiences are only a phase. In extreme cases, some sensitive individuals might even commit suicide because they believe their feelings do not matter to others.

Effects of Technology

Technology has exacerbated some of the difficulties teens face. It has changed how they interact with their world and even interfered with some aspects of their development. For example, teens hooked on technology may lack interpersonal skills and don't perceive social cues.

A 2018 Pew Research Center study found that 95% of American teens own a smartphone, with about half being online almost all the time (Anderson & Jiang, 2018). Social media and texting are changing virtually every aspect of teens' lives. The average teen uses a screen or device for around eight hours daily (Morin, 2022).

About half the teens surveyed were neutral about whether social media was negative or positive (Anderson & Jiang, 2018). Those with a positive view said it helped them maintain their connections with others and was a way to meet new people.

They also interacted with family members and like-minded people.

Nevertheless, social media has its downside. It can ruin offline friendships, change teen dating games, and introduce teens to shady people and sexual content online. Parents and teachers must explain to adolescents how to keep themselves safe online.

Social Interactions with Peers

Teenagers have complex social lives. They join new social circles and then abandon them. They fall in and out of love and face intense peer pressure. It's crucial for them to feel that they belong and fit in with other teens. It's natural for teens to move away from their parents and gravitate toward their peers—we see this in other mammals as well. Associating with and being part of a group is essential for survival. Loners risk death. There is a subliminal sense of urgency; teens experience this if they don't fit in with others. The need to belong is not something they decide on a whim because they are feeling lonely. This has been built into human DNA over millions of years (Dalai Lama Center for Peace and Education, 2014). Humans need social interaction—and teens must therefore be part of a social group. Numerous scientific studies on mental and physical health, longevity, and happiness show that relationships with others greatly influence these things and ensure positive outcomes.

If parents don't show empathy and understanding around the life-and-death situation adolescents face, this will make teens angry.

Hunger

This cause of anger is often overlooked. When blood sugar levels fall, teens become more emotional, unpredictable, and angry. Having something to eat and drink might be enough to overcome teen irritability.

Taking Away Their Things

Parents or caregivers should never take anything away from their teens as this makes them feel threatened—if they disobey, their parents will remove things they enjoy. Scaring young people doesn't guarantee obedience, although they might fear what will happen if they don't comply. Parents are supposed to care for their children, not frighten them.

Confiscating personal items can trigger a furious response. One teen recounts she became physically violent when her mother tried to take her phone or laptop, her primary means of staying connected at the time. Eventually, their relationship was so severely damaged that neither knew how to repair it.

High School Experiences

In the opinion of some teens, the U.S. high school system leaves much to be desired. While teachers in elementary school make the learning experience exciting and fun, this happens less in middle school, so students become unmotivated, and many need to improve academically. By the time the students reach high school, they often encounter teachers who have higher expectations and sometimes project their frustrations onto the students. In addition, some bored students start bullying others to relieve their feelings. This is why, in the opinion of some teens, the school system makes them very depressed.

One recent high school graduate advises teens on social media not to pay too much attention to their social status. "The moment these people are shipped off to college, all these cliques, social rankings, and BFF bully-squads will be dissolved, gone" (Kernan, 2019).

Around 5% of U.S. high school students drop out annually, so they may earn less over time than those who stay in school (Morin, 2022). These days, it's not only troubled teens who quit. Some burn out from the pressure of getting into a good college.

Bullying

Bullying has become more frequent. In 2019, 55% of American teens said bullying was a problem (DeSilver, 2019). Cyberbullying is also rising. In one study, almost a third of middle school respondents said cyberbullies targeted them in just one month (Scheidies, 2017).

Parents need to talk to their teens about these experiences, no matter how difficult, and explain when to seek help from adults.

Conflict With Parents

One of the teens' most significant conflict zones is their relationships with their parents. Situations that might provoke conflicts include

- their allowance and spending habits
- school and academic performance
- romantic partners, including public displays of affection and sex
- friendship choices
- cell phone use and time spent on social media
- chores and tidying up after themselves
- using electricity and hot water
- church attendance or religious choices
- clothing, hairstyles, personal hygiene, diet, and eating habits
- body piercings or tattoos
- curfew, transportation, and getting rides
- dishonesty, disrespect, and behaving unfairly toward others
- smoking and the use of drugs and alcohol

Depression

Around 17% of American teenagers, especially girls and mixed-race teens, are depressed at times (Morin, 2022). Seven percent of children aged 3–17 were diagnosed with anxiety disorders in 2016–17 (DeSilver, 2019). Too much screen time interferes with activities like playing sports, which can help ward off depression. Teens who frequently use social media might believe they are missing out, increasing feelings of isolation and loneliness.

Drug and Alcohol Use

Three percent of teens in the 9th, 10th, and 12th grades used marijuana daily in 2021, possibly due to changes in the law (Morin, 2022). In 2019, 51% of teens said drug addiction was a significant problem among their peers (DeSilver, 2019). However, the use of other substances has decreased.

Alcohol use and binge drinking have also decreased; however, in 2021, 26% of high school seniors still drank alcohol monthly (Morin, 2022). According to research by the Pew Research Center in 2019, 45% of teens said their friends were abusing alcohol (DeSilver, 2019).

Exposure to the News Cycle

News networks thrive on sensationalism, which often includes being the bearer of bad news. Teens who follow the news closely can become hyper-aware of adverse local and international events, including armed conflicts, natural and manufactured disasters, political instability, etc. This can increase stress and feelings of powerlessness, which can trigger anxiety.

Gangs

The number of gangs in schools dropped by almost half between 2001 and 2015 (DeSilver, 2019). Black and Hispanic students and those in city schools were most likely to report gangs at school.

Gossip

Gossip can be insidious and secretive. When a teen hears second or thirdhand stories about themselves, this can be hurtful, reduce their sense of self-worth, and might even provoke violence. Teens should be careful not to spread rumors about others.

Life Changes

Significant life changes like moving houses, starting at a new school, or family changes (for example, divorce or remarriage) can increase teen stress and anxiety.

Obesity

Almost a quarter of adolescents aged 12–19 are obese, with children of color more likely to be overweight (Morin, 2022). These children are more likely to experience bullying and risk developing severe health problems like diabetes, arthritis, cancer, and heart disease. Many parents appear unaware of their children's weight issues.

Peer Pressure

As children enter their teens, they start choosing their own friends and social circles and probably spend more time with their peer group than any other people in their lives. They compare themselves to their peers and look to them for inspiration. Most of all, teens want to belong, to hang out with people they—and others—admire, and to follow the crowd. There is a lot of pressure to conform, and it's hard to resist. Teens don't want to be left out. The downside of social interaction is that a teen might trade group membership or friendships for morality, which is peer pressure. Teens tend to be pressured into behaviors they might not normally do—like having sex, using drugs or alcohol, and bullying others. There is pressure to share explicit images and inappropriate photographs online.

Sexual Activity

Over the last decade, fewer teens had sex or were sexually active. Correspondingly, the teen birth rate has reduced, accounting for just 5% of all births in 2020 (Morin, 2022). Adolescents are, however, more likely to contract sexually transmitted diseases.

Traumatic Events

These may include abuse, accidents, bereavement, or severe illness. Other traumatic events might be school shootings, mass shootings, and other forms of violence closer to home.

Violence

Most teens will ultimately be exposed to violence in various types of media. Watching violence can decrease empathy and raise aggression. Parents need to monitor teens' screen activity, ban R-rated movies or M-rated video games, and avoid consuming violent content themselves. Talk to teens about what they are watching.

Some teens take out their anger by physically harming others. Once their triggers are identified and resolved, they will be calmer and less likely to get into physical fights. Teens might also experience dating violence, the effects of which can spread through their social circles.

TEEN STRESS AND ANXIETY

Teen stress and anxiety are increasing, and they are the primary invisible triggers beneath teen anger today. In 2017, the American Psychological Association determined that adolescent stress was becoming serious (Smith, 2022). School performance, getting into a good college, and deciding on a career path caused teens the most stress. 65% of teens were also concerned about their family's finances (Smith, 2022).

Several teens surveyed said they felt irritable, angry, nervous, anxious, tired, or overwhelmed. Some were short with classmates or teammates, with 51% saying that others regularly mentioned that they seemed stressed (Smith, 2022).

The Difference Between Stress and Anxiety

It's often hard to tell the difference between stress and anxiety as they overlap somewhat.

Stress is a reaction to a situation and is usually sparked by something external, like writing an exam. It might generate anxiety, but this is generally short-lived. Some stress and anxiety can motivate teens to improve or re-evaluate their lives.

Anxiety is a stress response rooted in fear, an emotional response to a perceived threat. Indications that anxiety is an issue are when vague feelings of unease persist, even after the stressor is removed, or the person continues feeling tense or worried. Anxious people often fear the future, expecting the worst.

If anxiety interferes with a teen's ability to live everyday life, help might be needed. Indications of anxiety include worrying continuously, irritability, and tension. Anxiety sufferers may experience insomnia, headaches, stomachaches, appetite changes, muscle tension, and pain. In extreme cases, it can manifest as obsessive thoughts, compulsive behaviors, and even phobias.

Indicators of Stress in Teens

Many teens are still experiencing some form of distress post-pandemic, especially if they are bereaved. Signs may include

- avoiding personal relationships, including online contact
- losing interest in activities previously enjoyed
- mood swings characterized by irritability, hopelessness, or rage and having continuous spats with friends and family
- changes in sleeping patterns
- changes in appetite, eating patterns, or weight
- losing interest in schoolwork and not being able to concentrate, think coherently, or remember things
- increased reckless behavior, including using drugs or alcohol
- thoughts or talking about suicide and death

Why Do Some Teens Struggle with Anxiety?

Any of the triggers mentioned previously could cause adolescents to develop anxiety disorders if they are not addressed. This is partly because normal emotions and stress responses may be unusually intense, especially in early puberty. Anxiety and panic disorders tend to manifest at that time, with girls much more likely to experience them than boys. This could affect every aspect of their lives. While being anxious is not necessarily attention-seeking, the behaviors it provokes do attract attention.

Signs that a teen is suffering from anxiety are much the same as those indicating that they are stressed—interrupted sleep patterns, nightmares, stomach problems, irritability, headaches, exhaustion, throwing tantrums, racing heart, and shortness of breath. Anxious teens constantly talk about their worries or fears, spend more time alone than their peers, or avoid social contact altogether. They often do poorly academically and might skip classes or school.

Causes of Anxiety

- Biology: If the nervous system is out of sync, some people could biologically be more inclined to be anxious.
- Environment: Stressful experiences and situations may trigger anxiety.
- Genetics: If there is a family history of anxiety, there is a greater chance of it manifesting down the generations.
- Learned behavior: Children will mimic the anxious behavior of the people around them.

Post-Traumatic Stress Disorder

Many anxiety symptoms mimic those of post-traumatic stress disorder (PTSD), which causes many teens to wonder whether they have the latter. However, the symptoms of PTSD can usually be traced to a particular event, whereas anxiety cannot. People with PTSD find it very challenging to recover from overwhelming experiences or form good relationships with others as their thought patterns are disrupted.

PTSD-specific symptoms include flashbacks to the event, avoiding anything that might seem related, feeling detached and emotionally numb, having negative thoughts, and experiencing anger, hostility, restlessness, sleep difficulties, and other symptoms that mimic those of anxiety.

Complex PTSD (C-PTSD) manifests when someone repeatedly experiences the same trauma. For example, a teen may present with C-PTSD after suffering a prolonged period of narcissistic parental abuse. Low self-worth is a key symptom.

People with C-PTSD also

- avoid situations reminiscent of the trauma they experienced
- feel dizzy or nauseous when they think about it
- are continually in a state of high alert
- believe the world is dangerous
- have trust issues
- have trouble concentrating and sleeping

PTSD is very complex, requiring personalized treatment. It's essential to find the right trauma counselor or therapist. It can also be helpful to have someone supportive, reassuring the sufferers that they are beautiful and worthwhile despite their negative experiences. Patience during therapy is essential. Being part of a community can help to create feelings of self-worth.

WHEN ANGER BECOMES DANGEROUS

Around 40% of teens experience anger; boys are three times more likely to have problems managing it than girls. Two-thirds of American adolescents have experienced such raw outrage that they have destroyed property, threatened violence, or perpetrated violent attacks (Rawhide Youth Services, 2015). Boys express this powerful emotion physically, while girls mostly verbalize their feelings.

As a parent, it's essential to differentiate between whether you have an angry teen or a teen who is angry. A teen who is angry will sometimes get angry, but the emotion will fade over time or once the situation is resolved. An angry teen will be angry about almost everything instead of just the occasional incident. Addressing perpetually angry teens is crucial, as only those who can control their emotions will become properly functioning adults.

Some indications that anger is a problem for your teenager include:

- Overwhelmed anger: This is sparked when your teen feels that they cannot cope with life's demands and becomes angry.
- Chronic anger: This never really lets up. It can ultimately compromise your teen's immune system and could cause anxiety disorders and depression.
- Judgmental anger: This is usually directed outward and might foster jealousy and resentment in others. Its hallmark is verbal abuse.

- Self-inflicted anger: There is a tendency to self-harm to relieve intense low self-esteem or guilt.
- Retaliatory anger: As the name implies, this is anger directed at people or organizations your teen feels have harmed them somehow. It can be destructive.
- Volatile or explosive anger: This dangerous form of anger erupts out of nowhere, is usually excessive, and can quickly turn violent toward others.
- Avoidant or passive anger: This may not be easy to detect and usually occurs when teens can't express their emotions.

Teens who are constantly angry can experience physical symptoms, such as headaches, stomachaches, trembling, dizziness, elevated blood pressure, increased heart rate, muscle tension, and adrenaline rushes. They clench their jaws or grind their teeth and might play with weapons.

If teens are always aggressively angry, they might get into physical fights, vandalize or destroy property, harm animals, and threaten others. This type of anger is a severe problem in America today, with 63% of children and teens manifesting some form of aggressive, antisocial behavior (Rawhide Youth Services, 2015). These problems can nearly always be overcome through anger management.

There are other problems with chronic anger. It might reduce opportunities as it steals the energy teens could use to establish their identities. Being angry might mean they miss out on physical activities that could provide a safe outlet for their emotions. Being perpetually hostile and tense ultimately affects their health. This is a tremendous cost for brief moments of fury about things that won't impact their lives much in the long term (Charles Hurst Reinvention, 2022).

POSITIVE ACTIONS TEENS CAN TAKE

Identify Your Triggers

It's vital to identify what triggers your anger. You might need to spend time alone to do this, but it will help you understand your anger and overcome negative behavioral responses. Here are three easy steps for identifying and understanding your anger triggers:

1. First, listen to your feelings and your body. When you start becoming overwhelmingly angry, stop. What do you feel besides anger? What is happening physically? Is your heart pounding? Are you breathing quickly? Doing this makes it easier for you to identify what happened to trigger this response.
2. Backtrack. What led up to you feeling the way you do? What were you doing? When did you start getting angry? It's okay if it doesn't make sense. You could be dealing with an invisible trigger, or you've been suppressing something.
3. Repeat the process. You might not be able to identify the trigger immediately. It might be difficult to unravel what happened or how you reacted. Keep going until you've resolved the issue.

How to Manage Your Triggers

Most people have dozens of triggers, so trying to identify all of them at once can seem overwhelming. You'll likely find recurring triggers once you've completed the above steps. Decide on the three most frequent or strongest triggers and focus on those.

When you look deeper at your triggers, consider the time of day and your physical state. Were you hungry, tired, or stressed?

Besides reflecting on what happened just before you started feeling angry, consider what you're telling yourself about that event. What others say or do is their problem, whereas what *we* see and hear—or think we see and hear—is about us and our response. Decide whether you're misinterpreting an event or something someone else said or did. Your interpretation of events or social interactions could be triggering your anger.

Your body might respond to the perceived trigger faster than your mind. What happens when you get upset? Does your face flush? Do you start shaking? Does your heart beat faster? Recognizing these signs means that you can control your reaction before it controls you.

When you feel these physical symptoms beginning, stop. Take deep breaths and focus on your breathing. Sometimes, it takes a few deep breaths to interrupt the cycle so you can notice what's happening and modify your response.

Do something. Get up, open a window, or make something to drink. If the situation is emotionally charged, leave the room. When you first do this, you might get angry. With practice, you can take these actions before your anger rises.

Thoughts lead to emotions, and emotions lead to actions. Notice how you start thinking irrationally as soon as you're triggered—things like "My mother doesn't respect me" or "My friends hate my hair." As soon as these thoughts enter your head, stop thinking and start breathing. This will defuse your reactions before they start.

You'll need to become more mindful when managing your triggers and anger this way. Notice what happens to your body and your thoughts when you are triggered. Find ways to calm down before you get outraged and say or do something you regret later.

3

GETTING TO KNOW AND LOVE YOURSELF

> *To be beautiful means to be yourself. You don't need to be accepted by others. You need to accept yourself.*
>
> — THICH NHAT HANH

The value of unhappy adolescence can be surprising. Commenting on a YouTube video, someone posting as Mariweem says they've finally realized that others will be drawn to you if you love yourself. "Just the simple act of smiling, and seeing others become happy because of my own happiness, is something I never dreamed was possible" (2020).

Anger and pain often go together. One of my friends once asked me how she could stop her teenage daughter from being so mean when she is angry; specific topics of conversation seem to trigger this behavior. I explained that these things are painful for her daughter to hear. When someone is feeling pain, they sometimes want to pass it on. Her daughter's meanness is her natural defense mechanism. I suggested she sit down with her daughter the next time this happens and discover why she gets so angry. What she finds painful to talk about are good examples of invisible triggers. It's like having a wound—a slight touch can be unbearable.

Your anger issues say something about who you are. Before you can deal with them, it is essential to know yourself.

UNDERSTANDING TEEN MOODINESS

Teens sometimes experience mood swings that appear mercurial, going from one extreme to another and everything between within days—and sometimes just a few hours. This can be challenging for teens and parents alike, as one never quite knows where they are on the emotional scale and how they will react to anything. There are several physiological reasons why this happens.

Puberty begins biologically when the hypothalamus in the brain starts producing the protein kisspeptin. This stimulates the pituitary gland to release reproductive hormones like testosterone, estrogen, and progesterone. These are essential for human sexuality and fertility as they regulate everything from menstruation and pregnancy to libido and menopause. Besides heralding puberty, they make teens susceptible to emotionally charged or risky experiences. As discussed, excessive hormones in the bloodstream can also make teens moody.

But there's another possible reason for adolescent moodiness. In response to stress, the brain releases the hormone allopregnanolone (THP), a natural tranquilizer. This differs from the fight-or-flight response and happens sometime after the event that triggered its release. It calms the brain, reducing anxiety and stress so the individual can function normally. Unfortunately, scientists find that the release of THP has the opposite effect on adolescent brains, keeping teens totally anxious (Swaminathan, 2007).

The Upside of Mood Swings

Experiencing and facing challenges during adolescence, like supporting your family, problems with relationships, and school or academic issues, can make teens stronger. This stands them in good stead when they enter adulthood. These challenges and struggles build their character, so they develop initiative. This vital characteristic can be very beneficial throughout life.

Developing Your Adversity Quotient

Until recently, it was believed that your intelligence quotient (IQ) determines your success or failure. This emphasized academic aptitude and performance rather than teaching young people life skills so they could successfully navigate life's ups and downs, which created both opportunities and setbacks. Being able to cope with difficulties and find the opportunities hidden in challenges and obstacles is known as the adversity quotient (AQ). Rising above one's circumstances and finding the silver linings in life's clouds determines success in life and at work. AQ can be developed over time and will improve personal qualities like resilience, courage, and persistence. Eventually, our mindset changes, and we become conquerors rather than victims tossed about in the storms of life.

Developing Initiative

Initiative describes the ability to move forward in life purposefully. Motivating oneself and finding ways to accomplish long-term goals are hallmarks of the initiative. This character trait develops in adolescence when teens form supportive relationships with adults. This is the main reason adults succeed in life, as opposed to intelligence or genetic predisposition. When initiative combines with kindness, empathy, and compassion, it becomes a positive character trait. Teens typically develop initiative when involved in projects that provide internal rewards, such as creative pursuits or making a difference in others' lives.

The Downside of Perfection

Adolescents should beware of falling into the trap of believing they must be perfect, as this could stunt their development. I was one of those teens. I was a straight-A student who always put a foot in the right place and behaved appropriately. The community believed I was a polite kid—and I wouldn't say I liked it. I never made any mistakes because I felt I couldn't afford to. I set the bar so high that I couldn't keep to it, and the fallout was hard when it inevitably came.

When you spend your life allowing others to tell you what to do, you never learn to make your own decisions or mistakes. You feel like you need more direction. The truth is that everyone makes mistakes at times. This is part of being human and can be the best part of life. Mistakes are the things we remember and laugh about later. They help us understand ourselves better and determine our belief systems. Mistakes reveal who we are at our core. Teens should be encouraged to test the boundaries and make mistakes, which means they know who they are and understand themselves better.

DEALING WITH STRESS AND ANXIETY AS A TEENAGER

One way to explain the effects of stress and anxiety is to compare them to holding a glass of water in the palm of your hand. If you hold the glass for a few minutes, it isn't particularly heavy. After an hour, your arm might start aching. After a day, your arm will feel numb and almost paralyzed. It's the same with stress and anxiety. If you focus on them briefly, they have little effect. But the longer you think about them, the heavier they get. If you focus on them to the exclusion of all else, you eventually feel paralyzed. What happens if we add more water? The glass gets heavier, and now you're worried about spilling some.

Imagine that your brain is the glass. If you keep filling it with stress and emotions and holding onto it, you start overthinking. Some of the water will evaporate, making the glass lighter. But if you keep filling the glass—or others do—it becomes heavier again.

The best solution is to put the glass down or drink the water. This will immediately make you feel better. You will start seeing things more clearly, and you'll be able to tackle the things that caused the problem. Sometimes, you think that dwelling on your problems constantly will help solve them, but that is often counterproductive.

Fortunately, there are things you can do to help you carry the glass and defuse your emotions without getting into a temper and upsetting those around you.

Meditation

Meditation is an effective tool for people to log off, manage stress, and rest their brains. It improves brain development while also reducing depression, anxiety, and stress. You can do meditation virtually anywhere. I'll discuss meditation in more detail in Chapter 6.

Exercise

Exercise can involve training for strength and endurance or doing aerobics, which increases your heart rate and general fitness. It can be as simple as walking with or without the dog. Walking about two miles each day is enough to stay in shape and enjoy the fresh air outside (Beresin, 2019). Exercise maintains fitness and releases feel-good hormones like endorphins. My friend's teenage son told me that after he quit cigarettes and started jogging for 30–60 minutes daily, he felt that his anger issue was resolved (Woodley, 2023).

Yoga is a relaxing, gentle type of exercise involving bending and stretching. It is an Eastern practice that blends body and mind. This reduces stress and promotes overall wellness.

Sleep

The reason some teens struggle with mental health problems could be as simple as the fact that many of them don't get enough sleep. A study on adolescent sleep patterns by the Centers for Disease Control and Prevention found that around 55% of teens who experienced problems like anxiety and depression got just four or five hours of sleep a night—or less. Only about 25% of high school teens who slept at least eight hours a night reported having mental health issues (Sparks, 2023).

Sleep is especially crucial in the teenage years when the brain is maturing. Teenagers generally need around 8–10 hours of sleep to function optimally (Gavin, 2019). Sleep might be difficult to factor into teens' busy schedules, but it's essential. Insufficient sleep might cause sleep deprivation, affecting their grades, concentration, and relationships. Insufficient sleep could ultimately lead to health problems, like obesity and reduced immunity, or cause depression.

Getting better sleep means going to bed at the same time every night and waking up at the same time in the morning. Regular exercise helps. Keep lights turned down low as bedtime approaches to raise the melatonin levels in the body (this hormone promotes sleep). Relax by listening to gentle music or meditating before bed. Turn off all devices, and don't use the phone for at least an hour before bed (Gavin, 2019). The bedroom should be comfortable, dark, and slightly cool.

Incidentally, people who sleep more are happier. A 2013 study found that Dutch infants were happier than American babies because they got more sleep—around 20 hours a night. Parents also got more sleep, with adults averaging just over eight hours a night (Acosta, 2019).

Creativity

Creativity can be expressed in diverse ways and provides an emotional release. There are several options. In addition to conventional drawing and painting, there's journaling, pottery, photography, scrapbooking, decoupage, woodwork, or learning to play a musical instrument.

Playing With Pets

Interacting with and caring for pets is a great way to experience the comfort and companionship of a loved animal, which promotes relaxation all by itself.

Socializing

Friends of the same age need to meet and interact because they are all experiencing the same things. Having someone to talk to prevents burnout, releasing feel-good brain chemicals. Socializing need not be just hanging out and chatting—doing activities together is equally effective.

Appreciating Nature

We're so tied to our screens that we often forget to appreciate the world around us. Whether it's a gorgeous sunset or the first blossoms of spring, there's a wonderful world out there. Being out in nature makes us feel good, so take time to appreciate the beauty.

Logging Off

It might not seem easy to log off and turn off the phone, but we must live in the real world too. Turn off everything for an hour or so a day so you don't feel the need to respond to anything. This will provide stress relief.

Maintaining a Positive Mindset

As humans, we tend to dwell on negative experiences. We need to generate positivity and focus on things we are thankful for. This means we will move from disappointment to gratitude and positivity.

The brain's left prefrontal cortex generates positive emotions. People feel better if there is more significant activity in the left front portion of the brain than in the right. If this continues, the brain changes, resulting in a more positive mindset. When people practice gratitude, their brains release more reward-related transmitters like dopamine. Their minds are also clearer.

Surrounding yourself with optimistic, hopeful people will improve your outlook, helping you see the world more positively.

OVERCOMING SOCIAL ANXIETY

Social anxiety is a specific form of anxiety and isn't a personality trait like being shy and introverted. It is a debilitating fear that makes interaction with others very difficult. Life is a constant struggle. Those who suffer from social anxiety might require professional intervention.

According to a sufferer, some signs of social anxiety include

- practicing saying "hello" while waiting for the person at the other end of the phone to answer.
- sitting in a crowded room where everyone is minding their business and being convinced they're all watching and judging you.
- being in a room by yourself, surfing the internet, is an ideal vacation.
- attending a party with strangers is the most stressful experience imaginable.

The causes of social anxiety are obscure, but environmental factors and genetics might play a role along with negative social experiences like bullying. Sufferers loathe being in crowded places, going to restaurants, and shopping.

There are several things people experiencing this debilitating condition can do to improve their situation. It might be challenging at first, so persistence is vital. It's like going skydiving to alleviate a fear of heights, but the best way to start is to face the fear and force yourself to become more gregarious. Interacting socially with others is a life skill. The more you practice, the more you will improve and the easier it becomes (Paritosh, 2021). If you challenge yourself to do something you used to feel uncomfortable about each day, you will gain a lot over time.

Let's use a numerical example to explain this. Suppose your skill level is one at the start, and you don't do anything to change your situation. After a year, your skill level will still be one. But if you work at it and keep improving by just 1% every day, after 365 days, your skill level will increase to 37.78. This means you are 37.78 times better than a year ago.

Here are six things you can do to overcome social anxiety (Paritosh, 2021):

1. Choose a social activity involving a group situation and make plans to attend. Before you go, write down any worries about attending and consider how realistic these are.
2. Set modest goals. If you have severe social anxiety, attend a smaller gathering. The important thing is to get started.

3. Learn an essential coping skill, preferably one you can use anywhere, to help settle you. Breathe deeply or visualize being in a calm place.

4. Learn how to start conversations. When people first meet, they engage in small talk. Once they find common ground, the conversation opens up. Say something pleasant, like complimenting someone on their outfit or the dinner they just made (but don't overdo it), the weather (yes, really), mentioning a mutual friend, or asking about their background or interests (people enjoy talking about themselves). It's important to appear confident. Stand or sit upright and make good eye contact without staring.

5. Learn how to end conversations. Conversations, especially with new people, often wind down by themselves, but sometimes, you need to finish them. Making an excuse usually works—saying you need to freshen your drink, that it's getting late and you need to go home, or that you've seen someone else you need to talk to are ways to end a conversation graciously. Tell the person you enjoyed meeting them. Practice your exit lines before you go to the social event so you don't need to stay in a conversation for too long.

6. After the social occasion, evaluate yourself realistically. What went well? What could you improve upon? How did other people respond to you?

Although it may initially feel strange, striking up conversations becomes easier over time. This is where new friendships blossom. There's nothing better than having a few special friends to hang out with, so think about the rewards when you feel nervous. And keep practicing.

A counselor recounts how he helped a girl who was afraid of being around others in group therapy. After learning some basic social skills, she interacted with other children. Not only did she find her fears were unfounded, but she also discovered that other children enjoyed her company. Social anxiety sufferers who venture out of their comfort zones may have the same experience.

SUCCESSFULLY NAVIGATING CHALLENGES AS A TEENAGER

Resolving challenges requires determination, persistence, and curiosity. Without perseverance, things might become over-whelming, and it might be tempting to give up. So, it is vital to keep the momentum going. Set a goal and do everything possible to achieve it. Do new things or try new ways of doing things, and don't worry about making mistakes. Keep the goal in mind, as this will provide motivation when things get tough.

Self-confidence is an essential character trait that teens can develop. Believe in yourself no matter what happens, and don't be swayed by others' opinions. Focus on the goal.

Life is challenging. There are times when people need to do new, unfamiliar things. Exercise patience—it might take time to achieve a goal. First-time failures are common, but it's essential to learn from any mistakes and persist. Katy Perry was dropped by three record labels before she became successful. Well-known entrepreneur Richard Branson was declared bankrupt several times before finding his niche. J.K. Rowling, who wrote the famous *Harry Potter* series, was turned down by publishers several times before she published her first book.

Develop the necessary skills. Do everything gradually to avoid becoming overwhelmed. Make sure that supportive people are available for encouragement.

LEARNING TO LOVE YOURSELF

It's happened to all of us. We look in the mirror and don't like the person looking back. It might be your appearance, but sometimes you are mean to someone and feel ashamed.

Perhaps you thought that a classmate would make a wonderful friend. You live in the same part of town, like the same things, and might have a friend or two in common. But no matter what you do, she doesn't respond to your overtures. She's polite yet distant when you try to start a conversation or give her something you think she'd like. It's hard when your preludes for friendship are spurned. You might start wondering if there's something wrong with you.

Many teens feel awkward about themselves, partly because we live in a very appearance-conscious, comparative age. We see beautiful people in the media or look at celebrities and feel we don't make the cut. This attitude isn't healthy and can take a significant mental and physical toll if it persists.

Self-esteem means feeling good about oneself. People with good self-esteem feel liked and accepted, are proud of their achievements, and believe in themselves. Those who are unusually hard on themselves, feel bad about themselves, and constantly think they're not good enough might suffer from low self-esteem.

When people focus on the good aspects of our appearance or character, we feel good about ourselves. The same goes for having friends who like and encourage us. However, when people are constantly scolded, bullied, taunted, or teased in a mean way, they can start thinking negatively about themselves. But it doesn't have to stay that way.

Building Self-Esteem

You are the only person who will be with you forever, so it's vital to love yourself. Avoid being overly self-critical and start seeing yourself in a better light. Change the voice in your head to a positive one. Here are some suggestions.

- Focus on your more agreeable attributes rather than your flaws. You're still beautiful and unique even if you're not conventionally attractive.
- Get to know yourself. Keeping a journal can be helpful.
- Treat yourself or do things that make you happy. Buy a bar of chocolate, have a bubble bath, go for a walk, or play with a pet.
- Learn new things. Start playing a sport, learn to play a musical instrument, or take up a hobby. Knowing more things will make you confident, and you'll like yourself better.

- Be with people who value you. Find supportive friends and be one for others too.
- Avoid focusing only on your problems. Think about the good things as well.
- Help a friend. Helping people releases feel-good chemicals in the brain.
- Practice gratitude to get perspective. We all have something to be grateful for—even if it was just the beautiful sunset last night or how good your morning coffee tastes.
- Don't judge others. You don't need to love everyone, but being critical and negative will drag you down too.
- Being perpetually alone and unoccupied can reduce self-esteem, decrease motivation, and lead to mental health problems. Volunteer, participate in face-to-face social activities, or start a part-time job.

BECOMING SELF-AWARE

Becoming self-aware helps people identify and manage their emotions. Self-aware people are more likely to handle their lives competently. This quality enables people to see how they perceive themselves and discover how others see them. For example, taking five of your best friends and thinking about how they see themselves will be very close to how you see yourself.

Unaware people may harm and hurt themselves and others. Knowing who we are and how our actions affect others—and ourselves—makes life easier for everyone. Self-awareness includes character traits, values, emotions, habits, and the psychological needs behind our behaviors. People also need to be socially aware to attune themselves to others.

Becoming more self-aware means delving deeply into ourselves. If you ignore things, you won't be able to change for the better. This takes courage and honesty but results in better mental health. It's also possible to track the development of your identity and character.

How to Increase Self-Awareness

Set Personal Values

What is important to you? Consider times in your life when you were the happiest and were making good choices. Do the same for times when you felt proud, fulfilled, and satisfied. Ask yourself what you were doing then, whether others were involved, why the experience was significant, and any other factors that made you feel the way you did.

Write down your top values. Work through the list and sort the values in order of priority. Look at your top-priority values and check that they fit in with your life and what you want to do in the future. Remember to check your values to ensure you make the right decisions.

Keep an Emotional Journal

Journaling is writing down your thoughts and feelings to understand them and yourself better. You can also release overwhelming emotions, particularly when stressed, anxious, or depressed. Journaling can help you identify the sources of your stress and anxiety; from there, you can start finding solutions.

Prioritize your fears, problems, and concerns. Identify your triggers and learn to control them. Counter any negative thoughts and behaviors. Remember to note down positive experiences as well.

Other Activities

- Be prepared to go on a journey of self-exploration and discovery.
- Look into a mirror and talk to yourself like another person. This reduces self-criticism and tracks your attention and emotions.
- Spend less time on your phone. People are becoming anxious, self-absorbed, and less empathetic because we spend less time maintaining face-to-face contact.
- Ask your loved ones how they see you in different situations. This can identify blind spots in your behavior so that you can improve.
- If you're angry, you might believe you have good reasons for your feelings. However, the experience might be quite different for the other person. Put yourself in their shoes. This will make you less critical and defensive and improve your relationship with them.
- Continually monitor your feelings and what might have made you feel that way.

LEARNING TO SAY "NO"

One of the hardest things for teenagers is to say "no." This is especially difficult when their friends or romantic partners try to pressure them into doing something they are reluctant to do. They want to belong, but sometimes, they can't go along with the crowd.

Peer pressure is when friends or other teens try to force others to do something they don't want to do because it makes them uncomfortable or might get them into trouble. Teens may worry they will lose friends if they don't do what the group wants. However, there are ways to say no without having a meltdown. Below are some suggestions.

- Teens can say "no" or "no, thank you" calmly and clearly without arguing. They should look the other person in the eye and stand up straight.
- They could provide reasons for their decision. If attending a late-night party means breaking curfew and possibly being grounded, for example, they should say so. They could add something like, "No, but thanks for asking me. Maybe next time."
- Turning it into a joke will change the mood, removing the pressure and attention from them. The others will probably stop insisting too.
- It often works to make an excuse. For example, teens could say they must wash the car or have an appointment to meet their moms. Anything will do.

- They could suggest doing a different activity, which gives everyone an out. Others might take up the suggestion as well.
- Teens can ignore the invitation and change the subject.
- Their friends might ask them several times. In this case, teens should stick to their decisions and not be forced into doing something they're not happy doing.
- Exiting the situation is another solution. Teens can make an excuse or walk away. One person's leave can inspire others, who may have their own reservations, to do the same.
- They could talk to their closest friends about their feelings and agree to stick together. This gives support to everyone.

EATING FOR OPTIMISM AND POSITIVITY

Parents do many things to ensure that their children are healthy and happy. Nevertheless, adolescents need to start taking care of themselves so they can do this once they reach adulthood. Everyone is super busy these days, but teens need to ensure their well-being.

You Are What You Eat

Believe it or not, the brain and gut are connected. The gut is lined with a vast network of nerve cells with millions of neurons. It contains more nerve cells than the combined spinal cord and peripheral nervous system. It's so extensive that scientists have nicknamed it the second brain. In addition, the gut has 30 different neurotransmitters that are also found in the brain. The gut produces and stores 95% of the body's serotonin, the "feel-good hormone" (Gerrie, 2020). The gut and brain communicate via the vagus nerve, a massive nerve linking the two.

Millions of bacteria and microbes live in the mucus layer that lines the intestinal walls. Since these microbes are located close to the nerve cells, they also respond via the vagus nerve when the brain indicates that the body is stressed, anxious, or happy. Signals move back and forth, with 90% of the vagus nerve carrying information from the gut to the brain, so the condition of the digestive system directly influences the brain (Gerrie, 2020). People with inflammatory bowel disease often suffer from depression and anxiety, for example. Certain beneficial microbes found in the gut stimulate the brain's production of GABA, a calming chemical.

Create good emotions. Every emotion gets stronger with regular use. Focus on your passion, excitement, and love such that positive emotions become stronger than negative ones like anger. People who experience a surfeit of good emotions don't respond angrily when upset. This is because their positive emotions influence their reactions.

Anger-Causing Foods

Did you know that certain foods can inflame anger in aggressive individuals? Trans fats stimulate aggression, while a lack of omega-3s in the diet increases the likelihood of depression and anxiety, which could make sufferers more irritable. Certain nutrient deficiencies can affect behavior too.

Foods likely to increase aggression and angry emotions include

- sweet treats—agave nectar (a sugar substitute), candy, and chewing gum
- certain vegetables and fruits, including eggplants, Brussels sprouts, cabbage, cauliflower, tomatoes, salads, and watermelon
- foods made with wheat, refined flour, and sugar
- preserved foods like cold-cut meats and canned foods
- dairy products
- greasy and oily foods like French fries and margarine
- snack foods, including salted peanuts, processed seeds (e.g., pumpkin and sunflower seeds), and dried fruits
- beverages like coffee, soda, and store-bought fruit juices

Teen Anxiety and Nutrition

Teen stress can manifest in several ways. Many teens experience digestive problems like stomachaches and constipation. A combination of stress and tummy troubles might cause insomnia. If there were nutritional deficits or tummy troubles during childhood, these escalate when children reach adolescence—teens need more nutritional support due to all the changes they are undergoing. Proper nutrition is essential to help them cope with stress and avoid developing full-blown anxiety.

Teens need enough zinc, which is involved in producing reproductive hormones, digestive enzymes, and feel-good brain chemicals like serotonin and dopamine. Zinc improves memory. Some people's bodies absorb less zinc when stressed, so it's crucial to eat a diet that includes zinc-containing foods (see list later in this chapter).

Vitamin B6 is another essential vitamin teens often lack. Besides creating feel-good chemicals like dopamine, serotonin, and GABA, vitamin B6 removes toxins from the body, creates red blood cells, and ensures proper metabolism and sound sleep. Supplementation might be required—this works well with zinc. This vitamin can be depleted during stress and by some medications, so consult a doctor about the proper supplementation and eat plenty of foods rich in vitamin B6.

Certain foods, such as those containing gluten, can fuel inflammation and irritation in the gut. Stressed individuals may remain in a fight-or-flight state, which makes it difficult for their bodies to cope with additional demands. Aim to eat a balanced diet and remove certain foods briefly to see whether things improve.

High-carb foods like pasta, bread, and sweets raise blood sugar and release dopamine. (There's a reason why teens love sweet things.) However, once the sugar high wears off, teens may feel even more stressed and anxious. Reducing sugar and carb consumption can prevent sugar spikes from affecting teens' moods.

Constipation reflects potential digestive troubles. Eat plenty of fiber-rich foods and vegetables and drink plenty of water to avoid discomfort and help improve regularity.

Anxiety-Relieving Foods

Certain foods are valuable for beating anxiety disorders and depression because they contain mood-boosting nutrients.

- Almonds contain loads of magnesium, making them a great anxiety buster. One ounce (12 almonds) contains 19% of the recommended daily magnesium allowance (Truschel, 2019).
- Asparagus contains folate, a natural mood booster. One cup provides two-thirds of your recommended daily allowance (Truschel, 2019).
- Avocados are rich in vitamin B6. As mentioned previously, many anxiety sufferers are deficient in this vitamin.
- Blueberries contain vitamin C, a powerful antioxidant. What most people don't know is that antioxidants can help reduce anxiety.
- Kale is also very rich in vitamin C and antioxidants.
- Salmon, chia seeds, soybeans, and walnuts are rich in omega-3 fatty acids. This helps maintain a healthy brain-gut microbiome.
- Turkey contains tryptophan, an amino acid involved in producing serotonin. Tryptophan also reduces anxious feelings.
- Yogurt containing live cultures is packed with probiotics, which significantly reduces anxiety. Similar foods include sauerkraut, kombucha, and pickles.

Nutritional Support for the Nervous System

Some foods strengthen the nervous system, especially the myelin sheath. This improves the communication between neurons, as discussed in Chapter 1. To feed the nervous system, eat foods that contain the following:

- omega-3 fatty acids (nuts, seeds, herring, salmon, sardines, avocados, and blackberries)
- iron (red meat, spinach, and broccoli)
- iodine (seaweed and iodized sea salt)
- zinc (red meat, poultry, seafood, nuts, beans, whole grains, cereals, and dairy products)
- choline (meat, poultry, fish, eggs, and dairy products)
- B vitamins and folic acid (chicken, beef liver, seafood, and eggs)

SUCCESS STORIES

Developing Positive, Helpful Thoughts

When LilyAnn was 16, she started seeing a life coach because she doubted herself. Her fear of rejection and failure prevented her from taking the necessary steps to fulfill her hopes and dreams. During the sessions, she realized that her negative self-talk was hampering what she wanted to do and become. As her awareness grew, she developed more positive, helpful thoughts. She learned about her inner qualities and discovered that she felt better when she focused on the positive aspects of her personality and goals. She began taking healthy risks, like trying out for the school play. She prepared herself and did not let her nervousness stop her from auditioning. To her delight, she landed a minor role. By developing self-awareness, she realized that she was strong and capable. She was also much happier.

Finding a Voice Amidst Chaos

Becca came from a dysfunctional, nomadic family. She was put into a children's home after her parents were arrested. Struggling with low self-esteem and bottled-up emotions, she initially found it hard to express herself, leading to peer misunderstandings. Therapy became her turning point. Through it, she discovered the nuances of effective communication, both verbal and non-verbal. A breakthrough came when she won a school debate, a testament to her evolving skills. Embracing her newfound confidence, Becca became a mediator among her peers, teaching them the art of understanding and being understood. Recognized for her abilities, the home's staff offered her an administrative intern role. Journaling one evening, Becca reflected, "From silence, I've learned the power of voice." Determined, she used her journey to guide others through their communication hurdles.

POSITIVE ACTIONS TEENS CAN TAKE

Start a journal so you can identify and manage your emotions better. This will improve your self-awareness and help you deal with stress, anxiety, and overwhelming emotions.

Tips for Keeping a Journal

- Set aside a few minutes every day for journaling.
- Keep a pen and paper handy to write down your thoughts anytime. You can also keep your journal on your phone.
- Write or draw whatever feels right at the time. There are no set formats for emotional journals. It's your private space, so don't worry about what others might think.
- Use your journal the way you want to. If you want to share it, that's fine. If you want to keep it private, that's okay too.

This will help you find order when life is chaotic, and you'll get to know yourself better as well. Writing in your journal might also be part of your relaxation time.

SUPPORTING TEENAGERS FAR AND WIDE

"You will not be punished for your anger, you will be punished by your anger."

— BUDDHA

Whether you're a parent or a teenager reading this book, you're here because you want to see a difference – either in yourself, or in someone you love. As we saw in the introduction, anger management is a skill many teenagers need – and it's not always something that parents and teachers find it easy to help them with.

I wrote this book to help with that. It became clear to me that more teenagers need this support than the few I'm able to work with directly, and it's my mission to spread this guidance as far as I can.

And this is where I'd like to ask for your help. I know you already have a lot on your plate, but don't worry – you can make an incredible difference without even leaving your home. All it takes to reach more people is to keep the conversation going – and to do that, all you need to do is leave your honest feedback online.

By leaving a review of this book on Amazon, you'll light a path towards the information and guidance that both parents and teenagers are looking for – and in turn, you'll

help more teenagers gather the skills they need to manage their anger both now and well into the future.

Reviews help people to find the resources they're looking for, and as I'm sure you know all too well, this is help that people want to find easily without having to spend a lot of valuable time researching the options.

Thank you so much for your support. There are so many teens out there who crave this understanding and support. Together, we can make sure they get it.

Scan the QR code below for a quick review!

4

DEFUSING THE BOMB

When adversity strikes, that's when you have to be the most calm. Take a step back, stay strong, stay grounded, and press on.

— LL COOL J

If teens know their triggers and change their perceptions, they will be calmer. When someone's desires or expectations aren't being fulfilled, this might cause angry outbursts. The only way to avoid this is to be happy with whatever we have and expect less of others.

Why do some things trigger us more than others? As mentioned previously, invisible triggers, in particular, are often based on negative experiences we had in the past. Based on past pain or hurt, our brains are wired to categorize these triggers as more threatening than they are. If a situation slightly resembles something that has previously hurt us, we can be triggered. It is our brain's natural defense. Everyone will have different triggers depending on their past experiences. These might include

- being excluded or ignored
- betrayal
- challenged beliefs
- disapproval or criticism
- feeling unwanted or unneeded
- helplessness
- loss of control
- injustice
- rejection

HOW DO WE KNOW WE ARE TRIGGERED?

We can instantly tell if someone has pushed our buttons when we feel an intense, uncomfortable, and often negative emotion. We might struggle to stop feeling it, even after the event has passed or we get new facts. Some signs of being triggered include panicking, crying, feeling overwhelmed, helpless, angry, or out of control. The person being triggered might react aggressively or defensively. They could have flashbacks to past events. They may withdraw or want to run away.

If the intense emotional discomfort lasts longer than a few minutes, what happened is a trigger. It's a sign that something in one's life needs work or support. An example of a trigger is someone who lost their parents in a car accident just before

Christmas. They might become sad and withdrawn whenever the holidays approach.

Emotional triggers often stimulate the body's fight-or-flight response. Parts of the brain shut down, so one will likely make poor decisions in the heat of the moment. It's better to wait until all the adrenaline and related chemicals have left the body before confronting the situation that triggered this response.

WHAT TO DO WHEN YOU ARE TRIGGERED

If it's a physical situation that's causing the problem, leave. Make an excuse or say, "I am feeling uncomfortable right now. I will catch up with you later."

First, select a calming action and try to relax (I'll discuss this in more detail in Chapter 5). Distract yourself by doing something you enjoy, like listening to music, walking, or running. Then, think about the event, identifying your thoughts and reframing them. Process your feelings (see Chapter 3 for guidelines). Having done all that—and only if you feel it would be helpful and are entirely calm—talk to those involved.

CONTROLLING YOUR THOUGHTS

It's easy to start imagining a worst-case scenario when something wrong happens or you are worried about something or someone. These statements rarely reflect reality. Some examples include thinking that you should quit school because you failed a test, deciding that you have worse luck than everyone else, or jumping to the conclusion that your friends have been in an accident when they are late.

Most people sometimes have negative thoughts, but it could be a problem if this happens regularly. These thought patterns may become a way of coping with adverse events or circumstances. The more prolonged and severe these thoughts are, the more frequently people might be inclined to think in this way.

Another problem with this type of thinking is that it tends to paint everything in black and white without allowing for shades of gray in between. For example, someone might think they are either headed for success or doomed to failure or that people are either angelic or evil. This is polarized thinking. Reality usually lies between these two extremes.

Look out for negative self-talk and reframe it. Here are a few tips:

- Identify the thoughts causing anxiety or dipping your mood.
- Intentionally look for shades of gray, alternative explanations, evidence, and optimistic interpretations of events.
- Perform a cost-benefit analysis. How have your thoughts helped you cope in the past? What are these negative thoughts costing you regarding your emotional well-being and relationships with others?
- Consider cognitive behavioral therapy. This teaches people how to identify, interrupt, and change their thinking patterns.

CHANGING YOUR BELIEFS

It often appears that external events cause our emotions, but it's our beliefs about a situation that make us react emotionally. Life happens, and our brains determine how to process and respond. Our emotions are, therefore, consequences of our beliefs. The good news is that we can change our thoughts, many of which may be irrational and have no basis. We need to differentiate between rational beliefs and irrational ones so that we can dispense with the latter. This will enable us to manage our emotional responses better.

This is sometimes referred to as the ABC model, which was developed by specialists in cognitive behavioral therapy. In this model, A refers to everyday life events, B refers to our rational and irrational beliefs, and C refers to the emotions triggered by B. If that sounds complicated, here's an illustrative example:

As a teen, if a friend says something mean to you (A), your initial thought (B) might be that they're trying to put you down. This could lead to a reaction (C) where you get mad and start an argument. However, by pausing and reflecting, you might consider that your friend had a rough day. Maybe they received a disappointing grade, felt overwhelmed by the feedback from a teacher, or had an argument with a family member before school, making them anxious about going home. Changing your thoughts and building empathy for your friend (a sign of AQ) instead of instinctively fighting makes you more supportive. As you can see, when B (your beliefs about a situation) change, so does C—your response.

LETTING THINGS GO

It's essential to learn to let things go. I've struggled with this myself. I've carried grudges for a long time, especially if someone disrespected me. Letting go is tough. The only way to do this is to move on and focus on something else.

When holding onto our anger, we tend to be self-focused, making it harder to let things go. When we can see the bigger picture or help others, we find ways to let go genuinely.

THE PROBLEM OF TOXIC POSITIVITY

Being angry doesn't mean someone is bad or broken. We are, however, responsible for what we do because of our feelings. Modern society frowns on specific emotions and people who are "out of control."

While focusing on positive emotions is good, we live in the real world where bad things happen. These unfortunate experiences can trigger negative emotions. When this occurs, beware of falling into the trap of toxic positivity. This is the belief that one needs to maintain a positive mindset regardless of one's experiences or situation. It's positive thinking taken to extremes. Toxic positivity invalidates or denies negative emotions. We must feel and deal with all our emotions to ensure good mental health. This could also be a way of avoiding another person's pain. In some circles, it is even considered gaslighting, making people question their feelings' validity.

An example of toxic positivity is when someone who has lost their job or experienced a bereavement is urged to look on the bright side or told that everything happens for a reason. While this might be intended sympathetically, it trivializes what the person is going through.

We can do this internally, too, dismissing or avoiding painful or uncomfortable emotions. Toxic positivity might stop us from facing our problems or ourselves honestly, preventing us from gaining insight into why we do things. This may hinder personal growth.

RESOLVING ADOLESCENT CONFLICTS AND TRIGGERS

Because they are developing on all fronts, teens experience frequent—sometimes daily—conflicts with friends and peers, teachers, parents, and other authority figures. Even minor disagreements might elicit disproportionate responses if these conflicts are not addressed quickly.

Conflicts With Parents

This is a significant issue for teens and their parents. One common real question many parents have is why they can't get along with their teenagers. When faced with a furious, yelling teen, it's difficult for a parent not to start sounding as though they, too, are adolescents. So, what's the answer to parent-teen conflict?

Listening Is Vital

Teens should give their parents dignity and appreciation, acknowledging everything their parents do for them. Teenagers also should remember to tell their parents they love them because they do beneath the turmoil. Good parents want what's best for their children, including teenagers (McKraken, 2020).

When conflicts arise, teens must listen to their parents, even if they disagree. They should see the situation from their parents' perspective and take their concerns seriously. It's best not to argue, as this might worsen things. Teens shouldn't yell at their parents—this might lead to a shouting match and won't resolve the problem. Instead, they should try and explain their feelings calmly and respectfully.

Parents must treat their teens as equals, allowing them to express their emotions constructively. Some teens feel that they need to suppress their feelings whenever a conflict arises—they are worried that if they cry or shout, their parents will explode.

If teens have done something wrong, they should take responsibility for their actions and apologize. This can help defuse a difficult situation and show that they are willing to make things right.

Dealing With Overbearing Parents

Some parents are overbearing—strict and controlling. Here are a few tips for teens in that situation.

- These teens must comfort and reassure their parents if they want more freedom. For example, a young teen I know and her mother each agreed to put trackers on their phones so each knows where the other is. She is at peace as long as the mother knows roughly where her daughter is.
- It's also helpful for teens to overcommunicate with this sort of parent, telling them where they will be, who they will be with, what their plans are, and when they will be back. Let them know if anything changes. By doing so, teens will earn their parents' trust and obtain more freedom.
- They need to show their parents things they would like to do or try as opposed to their parents just hearing about it. When, as a parent, I could see these kinds of things, I better understood the request and was more inclined to agree.

Dealing With Toxic Parents

Some unfortunate teens might have toxic or narcissistic parents, making life difficult. Toxic parents abuse their children emotionally, verbally, or physically. Substance abuse might be involved. These relationships begin in childhood and may continue into adulthood.

Signs of a toxic parent include:

- They are violent and physically abusive. This generates fear, anxiety, and anger. Violence has severe consequences and adversely affects relationships.
- The abuse might be verbal and emotional rather than physical. Children are belittled, emotionally blackmailed, called names in public, and humiliated. Their parents might gaslight them. This can be as harmful as physical abuse.
- Punishments are often harsher than the offense warrants, may include some form of abuse, and might even be dangerous.
- Such parents might be sexually inappropriate. This could include anything from sexual acts to exposing the child to explicit content. Parents who do this are in breach of the law.
- There are no boundaries; they ensure they are always the main attraction in their child's life.
- They take out their negative feelings on their children, leading to confusion and hurt.
- They become overly involved in their children's lives and so controlling that their children have almost no freedom.
- They expect their children to obey meekly and may become aggressive when their authority is questioned.
- Their needs are more important than their children's. This is a sign of narcissism.
- Their children must admire them. They become angry, resentful, and manipulative if they are not praised

constantly. This is another sign of narcissism.

- These parents are jealous and feel threatened when children develop close relationships with others. They might manipulate their children into ending these relationships or even end them for them.
- They don't support their children at all.

For teens in these situations, their lives become a nightmare of fear and defensiveness. They are traumatized and humiliated, and their experiences make them suspicious and hostile. They are constantly frustrated and resentful about their situation. Some lose track of who they are, and others develop mental disorders.

Tips for Teens Who Have Toxic Parents

- The utmost priority for teens facing these situations is their safety. If faced with physical abuse, finding a safe place away from the threat is crucial. Seek assistance from trusted adults, friends, or authorities, and consider not returning until there's a secure and supportive environment.
- These teens must focus on themselves, realizing that what their parents do to them reflects who *they* are, not who the teens are. They will then stop reacting to their toxic parent as if what was done was a personal attack. People who have good self-esteem and love themselves don't willfully hurt anyone. They don't need to bring someone down to feel better.

- These teens must set healthy boundaries depending on what's happening to them. These boundaries should be communicated clearly, even if others push back.
- These children shouldn't second-guess their feelings about what is happening. Their emotions are valid, even if others don't recognize them.
- Having realistic expectations is vital as this will reduce stress and avoid disappointment. Negative interactions won't necessarily turn positive.
- They can't change their parents—and they shouldn't try. They should focus on what they can control and change, like their own responses.
- Teens experiencing abuse must develop their own support network. This needs to include people they can contact about their problems and possible solutions. They could join a support group so they feel less isolated. Participating in activities enabling them to meet new people could be helpful.
- They must find a suitable outlet for expressing painful emotions like writing, listening to music, or reading.
- The situation will take its toll, so teens experiencing abuse must look after themselves. They could set aside a day each week to do something they enjoy to alleviate stress, for example.
- Teens with abusive parents should consider their future and plan to leave. This could involve getting a job, even a part-time one, so that they can support themselves. They should avoid their parents as much as possible.
- They need to bear in mind that they are not their parents and can make their own better choices.

- Teens can get help from the Substance Abuse and Mental Health Services Administration (SAMHSA) Helpline. SAMHSA provides free, confidential treatment, referrals, and information services for those facing abuse and its consequences. Their 24-hour hotline number is 1 (800) 662-4357.

Recommendations From Abused Teens

- When accosted by your parents, listen and ask for more information. Refrain from replying and avoid getting drawn into arguments.
- Half-agree with them and soothe them. This is called fogging and prevents toxic parents from getting their hooks into you. There is no reason to start an argument and create drama.
- Don't take the bait if your parents insult you with untruths or half-truths. Just tell them that this is their opinion and that you understand their viewpoint. Never be drawn into an argument or give them a reason to turn anything into a nasty scene.
- Focus your energies on other adults who are supportive and have your well-being in mind. Don't give in to your situation or give up.

Tips for Dealing With Sibling Conflicts

- Siblings must tell one another what is bothering them, expressing their feelings calmly and respectfully. Remember to listen to the other's point of view as well.

- It's easy to fall into a pattern of blaming or criticizing one's siblings, but this can worsen conflicts. Focus on the behavior or situation that is triggering the anger or frustration.
- Work together to try to find a realistic solution. It would help if you compromise, agree to differ, or focus on what you agree on.
- Siblings must respect each other's boundaries, privacy, and personal space.
- If the conflict is getting heated, take a break and return to the conversation when everyone has calmed down.
- If the problem can't be resolved, ask a trusted adult, such as a parent, counselor, or family member, to intervene.

Resolving Conflicts With Friends

The modern teenage definition of a friend is the first person who offers you a seat at lunch (Ruth M., 2018).

It's important to remember that even good friends sometimes disagree, argue, and fight. This is okay. If the friendship is healthy, conflicts can be settled. There are several reasons why friends might not see eye to eye:

- They may feel excluded, or there could be a misunderstanding.
- Their priorities might change.
- They end up having different interests and opinions.

- As their characters develop, they might have a personality clash.
- They may have different values.

Peer pressure can spark arguments if a friend doesn't want to do things the others are doing. There might be changes in friendship groups, and not everyone will get along. These things make friends feel disconnected. Friends might also have conflicts due to broken trust, bullying, manipulation, or competitiveness.

Tips for Resolving Conflicts With Friends

- Try to listen to one another and consider everyone's feelings.
- Be respectful.
- Keep it private—don't tell everyone about the argument or post it on social media.
- Avoid talking about the people involved; don't drag your other friends into the conflict.
- Don't try to get even or make impulsive remarks.
- If things get too heated, walk away. This will give everyone time to calm down. Use deep breathing. Try to talk things out when you feel calmer.
- After the fight, take some time to relax, then reflect on what happened. Ask yourself questions like:

  ○ What made you upset, hurt, or angry, and could you be overreacting?
  ○ Is it worth losing the friendship?

○ What do you want your friend to do or not do?

○ What bothers you most about the fight?

○ What role did you play?

○ How would you like things to be with your friend?

○ What might be happening to them to make them act differently?

○ Would it help to talk to someone outside the situation?

Conflicts with friends are typical in growing up, but they can be resolved with open communication and mutual respect. Teens can strengthen their friendships and improve mutual understanding by working together to find a solution.

SUCCESS STORIES

Turning Argument Into Encouragement

Anna is a high school student. Together with a few friends involved in a nonprofit organization, she volunteered to raise money to buy blankets for people affected by a Turkey earthquake. However, Anna and her friend Kelly disagreed about their fundraising approach. As the discussion progressed, the argument became more heated. They both raised their voices.

Other friends noticed what was happening and suggested they stop the discussion. Both teens went home frustrated and in a bad mood. Anna complained to her mom that her friend never took her suggestions seriously. After listening to her daughter, her mom asked what the goal of the discussion was. She explained that just because Kelly didn't agree with Anna's ideas, this didn't necessarily mean that she disagreed with Anna herself. Both girls worked hard to help others who desperately needed winter resources after a disaster. Then Anna realized she had become so caught up in her emotions that she had missed the bigger picture. Later, Anna and Kelly apologized to each other. They managed to work out a solution that everyone on the team agreed with and became closer friends.

Game Over—Or Not

Andrew enjoyed playing online video games but often became enraged while gaming. Once, he even smashed his computer monitors and hurt his hands. His parents were concerned and asked his school counselor for help. After a few sessions with Andrew, the counselor found that multiple things triggered the teen.

One was related to ego. Andrew would think something looked easy and begin bragging that he could do it. Then he would discover that these things were more complex than they seemed, and he'd realize he wasn't as good at certain things as he'd thought. He got mad and even accused other gamers of cheating.

Another difficulty with video games is that they are straightforward for children to access because the games are played online. Gamers in Andrew's group started making negative or inappropriate comments about his mother. This was another trigger for Andrew, who became very angry with other gamers when they did this.

The third trigger was that the video games had been developed rapidly without being adequately checked, so they were full of bugs. This upset the gamers, especially Andrew. While they were having fun, the games would suddenly stop working correctly, and the tutorials offered no solutions. This also sparked his rage.

Once Andrew realized what was triggering him, his perspective changed. He learned that it was not the other gamers' comments that made him mad—he allowed other people to affect his emotions. Andrew discovered the ability to let things go, becoming a peaceful gamer. He became a better team player and leader when he applied the same anger management techniques at soccer practice. After successfully passing the team tryout, Andrew joined the school soccer team the following semester.

POSITIVE ACTIONS TEENS CAN TAKE

Using the guidelines in this chapter, identify three of your most frequent emotional triggers.

Think about a few recent things that provoked a strong response within you. Write them down, then look at how you felt when these happened. Try to identify your emotions as accurately as possible.

Finally, replay the event in your mind. How could you have handled things differently? Was there a more constructive way you could have dealt with it? Repeat the cycle for each emotion you felt during the event.

5

EMOTIONAL CATCH AND RELEASE

 I gave myself permission to feel and experience all of my emotions. In order to do that, I had to stop being afraid to feel. In order to do that, I taught myself to believe that no matter what I felt or what happened when I felt it, I would be okay.

— IYANLA VANZANT

E ven if you do everything right, you will lose your temper occasionally. Your reactions are under your control. There is a magic action that can help you subdue your roaring emotions based on age-old wisdom and modern hand-brain techniques.

Our parents usually don't want or allow us to express anger as children and teens, especially toward them. This takes away our right to be angry and means we never learn how to communicate this strong emotion positively.

SUPPRESSING ANGER

Why do teens suppress anger?

- Parental or adult role models might have been aggressive and violent when angry, so their children never learned how to manage their feelings.
- Some youngsters are told they shouldn't complain, so they suppress their anger.
- Others may have witnessed violent anger, so they are afraid to voice their annoyance, frustration, or disappointment.
- If someone was or has recently been abused, bullied, or traumatized, especially if they couldn't express their feelings safely, they may still be nursing their anger.
- Anger might manifest faster when life becomes complex or challenging. It tends to leak out if it hasn't been expressed appropriately.

Anger is often suppressed because society teaches us that our emotions are messy and others can't deal with them. Unfortunately, when anger is subdued, it might cause a lot of hurt and break relationships when it eventually bursts out.

Suppressing anger may lead to anxiety, stress, depression, and feelings of worthlessness. The angry person's thoughts constantly whirl around the causes of their emotions—they second-guess themselves and overthink things. Anxiety and depression escalate. If this continues, the person eventually collapses or has embarrassing outbursts.

ANGER AND OTHER EMOTIONS

Sometimes, our emotions are so strong and overwhelming that it feels like our identity is wrapped up. This is especially true when we feel something intensely. But the reality is that our emotions are simply messengers. They provide information about our needs and our place in the world. We should notice and listen to them.

What Emotions Tell Us About Our Needs

Humans have two kinds of needs—physical and spiritual. Physical needs include basic survival needs like food, water, and shelter. We also need to be touched, exercise, and sleep, to name a few. Spiritual needs are more complex, and it's sometimes difficult to establish what we need. Our emotions help to develop these needs in our lives. These are friendship, belonging, harmony, beauty, inspiration, and peace.

Check-in with yourself regularly to establish what you still need to include. Do you need sleep? Are you hungry? Do you need to be heard or to feel safer? Then, consider what you might do to meet this need. Try to establish what your emotions attempt to tell you.

Understanding Your Emotions—The Emotion Wheel

Sometimes, teens might not have the vocabulary or communication skills to articulate their emotions, so eye-rolling becomes the prevalent avenue for many to convey their feelings. Most parents and teachers feel offended by this behavior. Introducing tools like the emotion wheel, which helps in identifying and expressing emotions, might provide a constructive solution. If you've ever attended art classes, you are probably familiar with the color wheel, a circle divided into segments where warm colors such as oranges, reds, and yellows are juxtaposed with their opposite cool colors like blue, green, and purple. Psychologist Robert Plutchik has created a similar emotional wheel that looks like a colorful flower with several petals. These petals represent different emotions and show how they can have varying intensities. For example, what starts as an annoyance can turn into anger. If not resolved, this, in turn, can intensify into a rage. Contempt or a tendency to aggression can fuel anger.

The wheel recognizes eight emotions—joy, trust, fear, surprise, sadness, anticipation, anger, and disgust (*Plutchik's Wheel of Emotions*, 2022). The goal of the wheel is to enable us to understand our emotions better and discover how to express our feelings more clearly.

According to Plutchik, these eight emotions are primary, each with a polar opposite, eliciting responses that are also opposites (*Plutchik's Wheel of Emotions*, 2022). For example, joy is the opposite of sadness. Psychologically, we are more likely to connect when we are happy and withdraw when we feel sad.

When it comes to anger, fear is its opposite emotion. Fear makes us want to become small and hide, while anger wants us to get big and loud.

Some emotions are a combination of two or more primary emotions. Anticipation and joy combine to create optimism, for instance. Joy and trust combine to form love. Emotions can be very complex, as discussed in this book, and breaking down feelings into their parts can help us understand them better.

The wheel of emotions demonstrates that emotions have different intensities. Boredom, for example, can intensify into loathing if left unchecked. The darker colors toward the wheel's center indicate the most intense emotion.

The wheel of emotions clearly shows that if we don't put the brakes on our feelings—or others don't—they will very likely intensify.

The wheel of emotion is a helpful tool for enhancing our emotional literacy, enabling us to understand our emotions and use the right words to communicate our feelings and the intensity thereof to others. It shows how different emotions are related and how they change, becoming more or less intense.

Dealing With Self-Criticism and Self-Judgment

When our anger is triggered, we might criticize or judge ourselves for our feelings. This complicates things as it adds more emotions to the mix. These may include guilt, shame, and anxiety. How do we stop this from happening?

- Emotions, as mentioned previously, are part of life. They aren't the enemy; they are part of what makes us human. Accept them.
- Step back and consider how the situation might look to others. This helps to establish the reasons for one's feelings.
- Be present without being judgmental, clingy, or trying to change the situation. This makes it easier to identify the emotions involved.
- We should be kind to ourselves as this stops us from overthinking our emotions.
- Those who criticize themselves excessively might be surrounded by toxic people, making things worse. In this case, stopping associating with them might be a good idea.
- Reframing thoughts can counter self-judgment and self-criticism. It is okay to have negative thoughts occasionally—you are human, after all.
- Avoid acting impulsively when negative thoughts descend. This could result in a downward spiral, causing more self-criticism if things don't go well.
- Finding better ways to manage our emotions enables us to avoid judging ourselves.
- By listening to our bodies, we can identify our emotions from the physical cues they give us before we do something that elicits self-criticism or self-judgment.

Your Emotions, Your Choice

When you feel angry, what happens next is up to you. You can choose to put the energy generated into something positive or negative. For example, reacting negatively—yelling, withdrawing, or lashing out—has some equally unfortunate consequences.

Negatively expressing anger can damage your health, as discussed previously. It can lead to social isolation because people will feel you are out of control. Being constantly angry might frighten others, especially if you are particularly aggressive.

Many teens resort to punching walls when they are furious. This isn't helpful. Not only might they hurt themselves, but it might also make them angrier. Every time they give in to their anger, they gradually change their personalities and become furious. The solution is to create more positive emotions. Correctly releasing this strong emotion is critical to avoid a vicious circle.

Yelling or throwing adult tantrums could harm the instigator and those around them. Angry people must know how to discharge the energy anger generates peacefully and constructively. Even though they might feel better after punching a wall, it harms their health as the body releases toxins during these episodes.

RELEASING STRONG EMOTIONS SAFELY

There are many ways of dealing with strong emotions like anger. Some of these are harmful, including denying or suppressing the emotion, withdrawing, bullying others, self-harming, and abusing alcohol or drugs. While some might be effective for a short time, they do not resolve the problem in the long term.

After avoiding acting impulsively and acknowledging all your emotions, consider how you can help yourself. There are several simple, constructive things you can do. Here are some ideas.

- Boost your mood. Being angry results in feelings of inadequacy, guilt, anxiety, or depression, so it makes sense to do a few things to improve your state of mind.

  o Play with an animal. This can be calming and will take your mind off your feelings.
  o Make a list of places you want to visit to generate excitement.
  o Read the story of someone you admire for inspiration.
  o Reorganize your room—a change is as good as a holiday.
  o Watch a funny video or movie.

- You might have identified some physical needs that are lacking. If necessary, have something to eat, drink water, shower, or nap if you are tired. Some people find that washing their face in cold water helps calm their anger significantly.

- There are several ways to reduce the negative feelings anger produces.

  ○ Punch a pillow, scream, or let yourself cry. All these will make you feel better.
  ○ Make a gratitude list.
  ○ Rip a piece of paper into small pieces.
  ○ Tickle a rubber band on your wrist.
  ○ Share your feelings with someone you trust.
  ○ Write a letter to the person who has upset you (don't send it to them).
  ○ Avoid using social media when you are feeling upset.

- Problem-solving: If specific problems were at the root of your outburst, consider ways to resolve them.

  ○ Talk them out with someone you trust and develop an action plan.
  ○ Make a list of your strengths without focusing on your current feelings.
  ○ When you are calm, talk directly to the person who upsets you. Explain what they did to upset you and how it affected you. Ask them not to do it again.

- Do acts of kindness.

  ○ Help someone you know or a stranger.
  ○ Volunteer your time.

- Take up a new hobby or spend time doing things you enjoy. You could

  ○ make a bracelet
  ○ read a book
  ○ sing or listen to music
  ○ go for a walk or run
  ○ play with Play-Doh
  ○ unplug by turning off your phone and other electronic devices for an hour or two (Mental Health America, 2019)

- Do exercises that promote relaxation. These can include

  ○ breathing exercises
  ○ progressive muscle relaxation
  ○ yoga or a guided meditation

- Ask for help. Speak to a trusted friend or adult or a counselor. You can also ask someone to sit with you.

Have a Go-To Release

We can revert to go-to-release if we are triggered or angry with someone or a particular situation. Besides those mentioned above, other strategies that are easy to do anywhere include emotional freedom techniques (EFT), trauma release exercises (TRE), and auto-chemical anger control.

EFT (Tapping)

Tapping is a technique grounded in the belief that emotional stress creates blockages in the body, hindering recovery and healing. It draws parallels to acupuncture in its approach but doesn't require needles. People can self-administer or tap on others. The process involves targeting specific energy points on the body, such as the center of the top of the head, just above the inner eyebrow corner, between the nose's base and the upper lip's top, between the lower lip and chin, about 4 inches beneath the armpit, and the inside of both wrists. Unlike targeting pain points, the emphasis is on energy points. Tapping can be beneficial during moments of acute anxiety or panic attacks.

The idea is to move the body out of the fight-or-flight response and into calmness and relaxation. Scientific studies have revealed that tapping releases stress and negative emotions while calming and regulating the nervous system. Tapping can also relieve depression and anxiety.

TRE (Trauma Release Exercises)

It involves deliberately making your body tremble to release old, buried stresses and tension. There's an effortless way to do TRE. Lie down on your back and bend your legs so your feet are touching but your knees are apart. Bring your knees together extremely slowly so that they start shaking. Keep your legs in that position so that the shaking continues.

Auto-Chemical Anger Control

When angry, I drop down on the floor and do 50 push-ups. If I am still angry, I do another 50. Usually, after the first 50, the brain starts releasing endorphins, which override cortisol, one of the stress hormones that create anger (Woodley, 2023). Use the energy your anger generates to enable these physical releases.

Doing this every time you feel angry will eventually train your brain to automatically release endorphins without you having to do the push-ups. Your body will do this whenever cortisol and other anger chemicals trigger your fury.

Anger—A Short-Lived Emotion

Keep in mind that the emotion will only last for a short while when angry. Based on my experience, remembering this has dramatically reduced the negative responses I typically have when I am angry.

Breathing Techniques

If you feel outraged and know that you need to slow down before responding to whatever has triggered or upset you, here are a few simple breathing techniques to calm yourself in the heat of the moment.

Breathe the Pain Out

Emotional pain often reveals itself in your body. For example, you may feel tightness in your chest if you are anxious. Breathe deeply, imagining you are filling the space where you feel that emotion lodging. It may feel that it's enlarging, but hang on. That's the breath or energy entering that space. Imagine the emotion leaving your body as you exhale deeply. Continue breathing deeply until the feeling peters out.

Hot Cocoa Breathing

Imagine that your hands are wrapped around a mug of cocoa. Breathe in through your nose as though inhaling that wonderfully warm, comforting smell. Then breathe out through your mouth for three seconds, pursing your lips as if you are blowing on the hot drink. Repeat four or five times until you feel yourself unwinding (Young, 2016).

Figure 8 Breathing

Draw the number 8 anywhere on your body with a finger. As you draw the top of the eight, breathe in for a count of three. When you draw the bottom of the number, breathe out for a count of three (Young, 2016). Do this slowly, relaxing while you breathe.

Other Options

- Write down your feelings. Ask yourself:

  ○ What part of me hurts?
  ○ What part of me needs healing?
  ○ What does this part of me want or need right now?

- Scream. This is a beautiful release; you'll feel much better afterward. If you're in a place where you can't let loose, you can make other noises like grunting, howling, sighing loudly, singing random syllables, screaming into a pillow, and shouting while you ride a bicycle. Alternatively, sit in a car with loud music playing.
- While you're screaming or making a noise, throw your body around.
- Dance to a strong beat, stomp your feet, or shake.
- Talk to the voices in your head. Imagine they are different characters. Listen to them and then let them go. This can also improve your self-image and enable you to decide whether these voices are telling you the truth.

THREE-STEP NPR ACTION

NPR is short for Nod, Press, Remind. This anger management technique has its roots in ancient Taoism. This Eastern religion arose around the fourth century B.C.E. and remains one of the primary religions in Eastern Asia today (Wikipedia, 2023). The symbol of Taoism is the well-known yin and yang image in a black-and-white circle. Taoism is a school of philosophical thought as well as a religion. They emphasize living in harmony with the Tao, which is the source of everything and underpins reality. Taoism has been the most important strain of Chinese thought after Confucianism through the ages and has significantly contributed to traditional Chinese medicine (TCM). The ancient Chinese philosopher and writer Laozi was Confucius's teacher and mentor. Wikipedia has ranked Confucius fifth among the most influential people in history, after Muhammad, Isaac Newton, Jesus, and Gautama Buddha (2023).

NPR is an organic, healthy way to get past the original swell of extreme anger when blood rushes to your head.

1. The first step is to nod slowly when you first feel enraged. This is a method taught by Taoism, and it instantly relieves these strong emotions. Philosophical Taoism holds that if you can nod, you admit that all things in the world are acceptable.

2. The second step involves pressing a specific point on your palm called PC 8. To find this point, make a loose fist. Notice where the tip of your middle finger touches your palm? That's PC 8 (see the diagram on the right in Figure 4). Press it slightly for about two minutes (DuPuis, n.d.).

3. The third step is to remind oneself of the hand model of the brain (Siegel, 2017). It is like what we did in the second step. If you look at Figure 4 on the right, pressing the PC 8 point ensures the thumb (the

emotional part of our brain) stays tucked in and works with the other four fingers (the thinking part of our brain). This connection is crucial for our well-being. But, if you check the diagram on the left in Figure 4, you'll see the thumb is away from the fingers. This means our emotions have taken over, and we're not thinking clearly. For teens, the big lesson here is to make sure we don't let our emotions run the show. We want our feelings (thumb) and thoughts (four fingers) to work together.

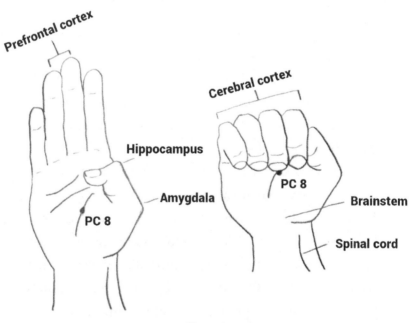

Figure 4

PC 8 is a unique point on your hand that experts in acupuncture and some doctors know can help calm you down. Think of it like a "chill button." You can activate this chill effect with techniques like deep breathing, meditation, or focusing your mind. Doing this, you're helping the intelligent, logical part of your brain (the prefrontal cortex) get back in control.

IT STOPS WITH YOU

Teenagers like to make their own decisions and may resent being told what to do. They often argue with their parents over seemingly insignificant things, like untidiness or messy rooms. Some teens with a particularly well-developed sense of self might insist on prolonging these arguments until they win, only to regret it afterward (RCC, 2016).

Teenagers and adults need to take responsibility for their actions when angry. Apologize to those you upset and forgive those who hurt you. Admit your weaknesses and reflect on your experience to see how you can improve your behavior.

6

JEDI MIND TRICKS

> *The more aware of your intentions and your experiences you become, the more you will be able to connect the two, and the more you will be able to create the experiences of your life consciously. This is the development of mastery. It is the creation of authentic power.*

— GARY ZUKAV

How do you react when you face insurmountable obstacles? Do you throw tantrums, sulk, or give up? Here are two inspiring stories of teenagers who faced significant life challenges and how they overcame them.

SUCCESS STORIES: FINDING YOUR ZEN

Finding Opportunity in a Setback

When preteen Zandra started using personal care and beauty products that her parents thoughtfully bought for her, she discovered that her skin reacted severely to nearly everything, from lip balm to body lotion. Instead of sulking and getting annoyed, she started making her own natural products that were kind to her body. Zandra then discovered that other people had the same issue, so she began to develop her range of natural beauty products and soon sold them at local farmers' markets. Her parents helped her start her business a few years later, and by the time she was 17, she was selling her artisanal skincare products as far away as New York (Winterboer, 2017).

What Zandra discovered is that inside every challenge lies a hidden opportunity. She not only runs her business, but she also donates a portion of her earnings to children's education. She has grown her business by surrounding herself with supportive friends and family and taking advantage of networking opportunities.

Calm After the Storm

Tennis champion Roger Federer wasn't always as calm and collected on the court as he is now. When he was younger, the tennis star had a significant problem—he revealed his anger very publicly at the world's best-known tennis tournaments. His outbursts were fueled by pressure, stress, and frustration.

He was disqualified from several tournaments. On one occasion, he hurled his racket so hard that it broke a heavy-duty curtain between two tennis courts. Not only was he disqualified, but he was also forced to do menial work. Federer had always been a hothead, even as a child, and didn't take kindly to discipline. His coaches quit, despite the tennis player's promise and ability. Nevertheless, his outbursts continued.

In his late teens, he eventually consulted a sports psychologist, looking for ways to tame his aggression. Therefore, his transition into today's Mr. Cool began. Always inclined to be emotional, it took him a few years to get his feelings under control, both on-court and off. Federer has spent years learning to channel his passionate emotions, and now they rarely get the better of him—although he will sometimes cry after winning a tough match.

MINDFULNESS FOR ANGER MANAGEMENT

Anger management is a skill that needs to be practiced even when you don't feel angry. The question is whether anger generates happiness and joy or improves your health. The answer is inevitably "no," so the next question is why people keep allowing their anger to control them.

If you regularly lose your temper or become enraged, you must acknowledge that you have a problem. This enables you to reflect on your triggers and reactions and determine how to avoid exploding when life happens.

Mindfulness is the key to listening to your anger rather than being its messenger. Anger management is a long process with self-mindedness at its core. First, establish how often you get angry. The answer might surprise you. The best way to do this is to "hammer a nail." Carry a small notebook with you and draw a short line whenever you get angry. This enables you to become more aware of when and how often you feel this strong emotion. Thus, being enlightened will make it easier to subdue your anger before you act on it.

Having done this, tell your family and friends what makes you angry. Do this tactfully so they don't feel they are to blame for your emotional problems. Aim to have peaceful, constructive conversations with them.

Learn how to articulate what is bothering you as soon as you feel angry when someone upsets you. Say things like, "I'm sorry, but I'm feeling kind of annoyed right now. It's making me anxious and a little irritated. I think it's about me and not you, so let me deal with that for a while."

Write down your experiences with anger in your emotional journal so you can reflect on what's happening and communicate with yourself. Therapists recommend this as it helps to put the noise in one's mind into words. Many people find that just doing this is enough to relieve the pressure of their feelings.

What Is Mindfulness?

As most people do, mindfulness enables us to achieve and maintain a greater awareness of ourselves rather than living on autopilot. This cultivates a conscious awareness of our thoughts, emotions, bodies, and world. Derived from Buddhism, mindfulness is an excellent way to manage stress and our emotional responses to our environments.

Mindfulness means separating ourselves from our thoughts, especially those that are negative, judgmental, or painful. If you get into the habit of observing your thoughts, you will see that many have little substance and are generally unhelpful. In the same way, we can perceive ourselves and our bodies. We don't need to identify with our thoughts, emotions, or bodies—these don't define us and don't make us who we are.

We need to accept our emotions without agonizing over the way we feel. Allow the feelings to play out and fade away as they naturally do. Mindfulness means being present in the current moment. Our thoughts include the past and future, and this generates more emotion. Focusing on your breathing, what you're experiencing through your senses, and being in tune with your body can also help ground you in the present.

Benefits of Mindfulness

Mindfulness has many mental health benefits. Studies indicate it can help practitioners manage stress and anxiety, reduce depression, and cope with serious illnesses. Consciously becoming mindful improves self-esteem and relaxation, producing more incredible zest for life in general. It changes brain regions associated with emotion, memory, and learning. One researcher found that it may also help young people by reducing stress, anxiety, and

hostility, leading to fewer arguments and better relationships.

DEVELOPING MINDFULNESS

We can become more aware of what's happening inside and
outside of us in several ways and learn to let go of things that
impede our progress.

Meditation

The practice of meditation dates back thousands of years and is
often coupled with spirituality. It's a way of focusing one's
mind or deepening awareness for a short period.

To meditate, find a quiet place away from distractions. Turn off
your phone and other devices and unplug while you are meditating. Choose a quiet time of day, such as very early in the
morning before family and work or school commitments
intrude. You could also meditate late at night or if you have a
regular quiet spell during the day.

Set the alarm so you don't need to worry about the time or
anything you need to do after you finish. Start with short
sessions of about five minutes and gradually extend these by 5–
10 minutes until you meditate for 30 minutes at a time (Cherry,
2022).

Prepare to meditate. Make sure that you are physically
comfortable. It would be best if you weren't too warm or too
cold. Hunger, thirst, and tiredness can be distractions, so make

sure you are none of these before you start meditating. You can sit in a chair or lie down.

General Mindfulness Meditation

Start with a full body scan. Focus on your entire body, from your head to your feet. Notice if you have any pain, tightness, or unusual sensations. Observe them without judging or feeling you need to do something about them.

Then, focus on your breathing, becoming aware of the process. Listen to the breath going in and out of your body. Let your thoughts come, and don't ignore or suppress them. Notice them, stay calm, and use your breathing as an anchor. If you start feeling anxious, worried, frightened, or hopeful, let the emotions go. This is very normal. Continue to focus on your breathing.

Sensory Exercises

Sensory activities can help focus the mind so that you do not dwell excessively on your thoughts or emotions. Here are a few activities suitable for teenagers:

- Carry a stress ball or pop it fidget toy to keep your hands busy.
- Do heavy work, including laundry, taking out the trash, washing cars, gardening, etc.
- Take a car, bus, train, or other transport—the motion is calming for some individuals.

- Cook—or learn how to—and notice the sensory experiences of taste, touch, texture, and temperature.
- Create a meal that features several flavors and textures.

Keeping Your Mind in the Present

Focusing on the present without worrying about the future or dwelling on the past is essential. In modern society, we're in a constant state of one or the other, which means we rarely notice or enjoy the present we live in. Here are some ways to become more present:

- Notice your environment. Close your eyes, take a deep breath, open your eyes, and look at where you are now. Notice the walls, floor, ceiling, windows, and lights. What do they look like, what color are they, and how many are there (in the case of windows and lights)?
- Do one thing at a time so you don't get overwhelmed. Multitasking can add to your workload and stress and reduce efficiency. Give your current task your undivided attention. Avoid the temptation to check your phone or indulge in other distractions.
- Gratitude for what you have now is vital for mindfulness and prevents us from longing for anything we don't have, such as relationships, material things, or qualifications. Write a list of what you are grateful for and update this daily. You'll be amazed at how good your life is.
- Accept things the way they are. Let go of how you imagined they would be or how you would like them to

be. Sometimes, things don't work out the way you hoped they would.

- Surround yourself with positive, supportive people—and provide them with support and assistance when needed. You'll be surprised what a difference this makes.
- Be mindful in everything you do. When brushing your teeth, for example, focus on the toothpaste's taste, the brush's sensation in your mouth, and the temperature of the water. Chew a meal properly and enjoy the smell, flavors, and texture of the food.
- Practice deep breathing and meditation, as mentioned previously.
- Take a break from social media and technology, as these are very distracting and can prevent you from living in and enjoying the present moment. While you might think technology connects you to the world, very often, it's divorcing you from the one you live in.
- Get regular exercise or walk in a park or your local neighborhood to raise your awareness of where you are. Note the sounds, sights, and smells you experience on your walk.

SUCCESS STORY: CHORES AND PRIVILEGES

A mother had a problem with her 12-year-old daughter. The daughter would shout "No!" and verbally abuse her mom whenever she was asked to do something. The mother tried several strategies to get her daughter to comply, but the situation continued. The mother also began getting angry, and eventually, the two were experiencing constant shouting matches and heated exchanges. As you would expect, their relationship deteriorated.

Eventually, they decided to consult a life coach. The mother changed her strategy. She told her daughter to do only one thing at a time and stopped reminding her to do chores or warning her if she didn't. After telling her daughter what she wanted her to do, the mother would walk away immediately, ignoring her daughter's response. If the daughter didn't complete the task, one of her privileges was removed. Whenever her daughter tried to argue, the mom would walk away.

It didn't take long for the daughter to change her behavior. There were no more angry outbursts and blowups. Mom is less stressed, the daughter is doing what she has been asked to do, and the two have a better relationship.

7

ADULTING TEENAGERS

> *The young always have the same problem—how to rebel and conform at the same time. They have now solved that by defying their parents and copying one another.*
>
> — QUENTIN CRISP

Most parents want good relationships with their teens and cannot understand why this is so difficult. To find solutions, I interviewed many teens and parents. This chapter summarizes the ideal behaviors of parents from a teen's perspective and how parents would like their teens to relate to them and behave. Some of this chapter is based on the views of adults when they look back on their teenage years and consider what they wished they knew when they were that age.

One of the reasons for these relationship difficulties is that switching parenting styles can be challenging. When children are younger, they need their parents to decide for them. However, once they reach their teens, children want and need to make their own decisions, even if they are not the best. This is part of taking responsibility for themselves and is an essential step on their journey to adulthood. However, it can make parents feel superfluous. In addition, they might sometimes have differing views on their teens' decisions.

The irrational behavior of a teenager can leave parents feeling that they've entered an emotional minefield. One of the goals of adolescence is for young people to establish their own identities by discovering who they are and what role they might play in the adult world they will one day inhabit. They question everything, developing new opinions and worldviews. They evaluate everything—their gender, faith, intellect, and relationships. Their peers, especially those who seem more mature and confident, are their role models.

The mood swings and emotional turmoil teens experience can sometimes make their parents feel they're returning to the terrible twos. In both cases, the underlying reality is that children ultimately need to separate from their parents. While this is normal, especially during adolescence, the trouble with teenagers is that they are apt to make spur-of-the-moment decisions that could have severe consequences in the real world, whether these relate to friendships, school, activities, using drugs or alcohol, or having sex. This can make it difficult for parents to achieve a balance or intervene when their teens feel this is warranted.

There is, therefore, a certain inevitability to quarreling between parents and teens, but it doesn't mean the relationship is over if they do. Sometimes they will be comfortable together, doing everyday things and sharing experiences. Teens want recognition and respect from their parents they still love—and who love them too.

Teens want to be validated. When arguments between parents and their adolescent offspring flare up, they appear to be about superficial issues—a messy bedroom, a chore not done, or their curfew. Teens want their parents to acknowledge their maturity, capability, and, above all, their value as a person. For example, teens get annoyed if their parents say they can't go out on a school night. They may feel their parents don't trust them to make their own good decisions.

If teens' peers and friends check that they have everything they need when preparing to go out, they value this input and will accept it. However, when concerned parents do the same, they see an unintended subtext: they can't look after themselves. Because this might reflect some of their doubts about themselves, they might get annoyed, ignore the parent, or act as though they are indifferent.

PARENTS VERSUS TEENS—ANGER TRIGGERS FROM A PARENT'S PERSPECTIVE

The relationship between many parents and their adolescents may resemble a power struggle. Parents want to raise mentally and physically healthy adults who are responsible people capable of making informed choices. Unfortunately, their children are prone to impulsive decisions and poor choices at this time. On the other hand, teens yearn to have the independence and perceived freedom of adults but can't always appreciate the potentially negative consequences of their actions.

A significant amount of parent-teen conflict occurs because there is a big world out there, the potential of which excites adolescents, whose developing brains are inclined to portray new opportunities in rosy colors. Teens itch to explore the world. They sometimes deliberately make poor choices to get the desired experiences, even if they know the risks. They might then express their desires by becoming angry. The anger appears irrational to others, but teens may feel that there is no other way to explain their needs except doing something they know is incredibly stupid. This is very difficult to deal with as a parent because, as mentioned previously, the teen's dopamine center is being triggered by the promise of a new adventure—even if it will probably have a negative outcome.

Based on brain theory, the development of the brain during adolescence plays a big part in parental alienation. Teens are constantly disconnected from their parents because their emotions override rationality. All parents want to do is help. However, teens tend to interpret helpful gestures in the worst possible way.

Teens wonder why their parents get so annoyed over what they perceive as small things. They wonder if it matters that they got some dirt on the floor or forgot to put their shoes away or take out the trash. The parent, conversely, can't understand why their teen won't do what they've asked them to do several times. If a teen comes home yet again with a bad grade in a particular subject, parents might suggest extra tutoring so he can improve. However, the teen takes this as a personal affront. He knows he is doing poorly but fears his parents think he is stupid when all they want to do is help.

It never occurs to young children that their parents aren't perfect. When they become teenagers, however, they stop hero-worshiping their elders. They perceive their parents as equals, even while they are the leading authority figures in the teen's life. They see that their parents are real people with work difficulties, unappreciative spouses, and health problems. They might observe that a parent is rude and stingy to servers at a busy restaurant or that they go out of their way to help others in difficulty. Arguing becomes easier because teens suddenly realize that adults are imperfect human beings and they can be wrong.

Parents must resist the urge to join in the mudslinging if teens have a bad attitude. A neutral, matter-of-fact tone is best when establishing safe boundaries or rules. Teens are more likely to respond to this in an adult manner. Avoid speaking to teens as if they are young children, as this will infuriate them, and you will be less likely to get their cooperation.

Parents need to model appropriate behaviors, especially when managing their emotions, mirroring what they expect from their teens. If parents are struggling to talk about their feelings, they shouldn't hide them. If parents need therapy, they should tell their teens. This demonstrates that having emotional difficulties and asking for help when necessary is okay. If parents do deep breathing or meditation when angry, their teens may mimic them.

Although teens' raging hormones underlie their angry outbursts and mood swings, as a parent, you can get beyond this if you sit down with them. Respect them and try to explain your views without being demanding. Find the time when you can give one another your complete attention. You can't resolve issues when everyone is rushing around getting ready for school or work or when you get home exhausted.

Teenagers' parents must be good, empathetic listeners, as teens often feel that others don't understand them. Parents need to allow their teens to express their emotions and give them complete attention when they do. This will prevent teens from feeling vulnerable and misunderstood and reduce their angry responses. If anger threatens to boil over, parents should set some ground rules and decide on suitable punishments if they are not adhered to. This should be done in an unemotional way.

Another factor affecting parent-teen relationships is the general stress of running a household increases when teenagers inhabit it. Teens are very energetic, busy individuals. The change in tempo tends to happen gradually, so no one realizes how the stress is building up. This means the situation isn't addressed until everyone is on edge, which may result in more conflicts and arguments.

Parents should never compare their teenagers to other teens or adults. They hate this, and they will become stressed, angry, and uncooperative. They want to be valued for themselves and feel that they are enough.

Young people develop a sense of privacy during adolescence. It's essential that parents respect this at all costs. Suppose parents see signs that their teens might be getting violent, abusing alcohol or drugs, or engaging in risky and potentially dangerous behaviors. In that case, they might be tempted to disrespect their teens' privacy. Never do this; it could reduce their trust or ruin the relationship altogether if it is already on shaky ground. Treat them as you would an adult in this situation.

Don't judge their friendship choices. However, parents should intervene if it's something alarming. Romantic relationships can be an emotional roller coaster for teens. Experiencing conflicts or rejection can trigger feelings of anger and resentment. Be supportive when this happens.

AUTHORITATIVE PARENTING: THE BEST PARENTING STYLE

Often, it appears to adolescents that the adults in their lives are being hypocritical: They can do things, but their children can't. Because this is the time when teens question everything, this is another bomb waiting to explode. Even in today's more permissive society, many parents believe that they don't need to explain their decisions and that their teens should obey them without question. Teens are naturally inclined to rebel against this attitude. They intuitively know that if a parent can't explain the reason for a particular rule, they won't understand why they are enforcing it. In a sense, this is an abuse of parental authority. Demanding obedience in this fashion does not teach teens how to resolve conflicts or make compromises, and it won't earn their respect.

Treat teens as young adults while ensuring safe boundaries. Parents should tell their teens why they have made a particular rule or decision. Don't control them excessively or micro-manage every aspect of their lives, as they detest this; it makes them feel disempowered and could lead to conflict. Find ways to allow them to feel special. Let them choose their hair color and makeup, for example.

What Is Authoritative Parenting?

You might have heard of this parenting style, which is highly recommended. It's believed to be one of the best ways of raising children. Also known as democratic parenting, parents use reasoning and discussion with their children instead of expecting and enforcing blind obedience. Authoritative parenting is based on both high expectations and high responsiveness. These parents remain warm and responsive while setting high standards for their children.

This parenting style usually creates the best outcomes. Children raised this way are happy. They achieve more academically. They are independent and self-reliant. They have good self-esteem, can hold their own socially, and are warm, positive individuals. They regulate their emotions and have self-control. They have better mental health and are less likely to suffer from anxiety and depression, attempt suicide, or abuse alcohol and drugs.

Traits of authoritative parents include being warm, connected, and nurturing. They listen to their children and reason with them. They encourage autonomy and independence while at the same time setting clear boundaries and good behavioral rules. They use positive disciplinary techniques instead of forceful, punitive measures when children or teens transgress. They avoid trying to control their children by using psychological weapons like manipulation and threats. These parents tend to earn respect rather than insist on it.

CREATING WIN-WIN SITUATIONS

Rewards and Consequences

Parents can set up a system of rewards and consequences so their teens listen to them or behave responsibly without them having to yell. Good behavior is rewarded, while bad behavior brings uncomfortable results. These should be discussed with teens beforehand. The idea is for adolescents to make their own choices and learn to live with them. Positive reinforcement of good behavior often gets far better results than screaming and shouting when children misbehave.

Partnering With Teens

People can become better parents by partnering with their teens. Many parents ask questions that shame teens, like, "What's wrong with you?" Others might go to the opposite extreme, coddling them by sorting out their problems or giving

144 | SASHA WOODLEY

them material things in exchange for compliance. Instead, parents can use empathetic statements to connect with their teens. They could say, "You look like you had a rough day. If you'd like to talk about it, I'm here."

Story: A Recipe for Success

A mother went to a life coach, concerned about her teenage daughter, Jami, struggling with depression and anxiety. She had been self-harming and suicidal at times. When they went to the coach, they were practically enemies. The mother would take away Jami's phone, prevent her from seeing her friends, and sometimes have her locked down. The coach started by telling them they had to agree to negotiate and communicate their wants and needs. They should also tell one another what they want the other person to work on.

The coach suggested that Jami be rewarded for her efforts by earning back her privileges, which she would do after a set period. He also recommended that her mom allow her some phone time each day, even before Jami had honored their agreement. Jami agreed to her mom's terms. When her mother saw that Jami was ready to do that, she agreed to some of her daughter's terms. They also decided on the consequences if Jami didn't stick to her end of the agreement. Jami could choose which consequence she would prefer if she transgressed any rules. They also decided that if Jami broke a rule for several weeks, her mother got to choose the consequences. Her mom realized that if she didn't stick to her end of the agreement, she might lose Jami's trust—a mom's worst fear. Jami understood that if she did what her mother wanted, she would get all the desired freedoms, although she would need to earn them.

This ultimately healed the relationship between Jami and her mom. Not only that, Jami learned some valuable life skills. When she prepared to move out before college, her mother knew she could trust her daughter to make the right choices.

TIPS FOR COMMUNICATING WITH TEENS

Parenting teens isn't easy. As a parent, you may sometimes feel that your good intentions seem to be doing more to complicate or harm the relationship than to foster it. Your teen's behavior and refusal to take what you believe to be good advice may be frustrating and concerning. Maintaining a good relationship with your teen comes down to communication. Here are some tips for better communication.

- This can't be emphasized enough: Listening is essential. Don't question your teen directly about their day or other aspects of their lives; they might interpret this as interference and shut down. Instead, let them talk of their volition and listen to what they say. You will glean much information about what is happening in their lives this way. Stay open and interested, but be careful not to pry.
- Validate their feelings and show empathy. For example, avoid seeming judgmental or dismissive when your teen shares a disappointment with you. Instead of saying, "Well, they weren't right for you anyway," you

could say, "Wow, that sounds difficult." This will encourage your teen to open up more when speaking to you.

- Show that you trust them. Take your teen seriously. Ask them to do you a favor or put them forward for a privilege. This shows that you think they are capable and responsible. It will build their confidence in themselves and their abilities.

- Set the rules, but don't be a dictator. Be prepared to explain the reasons for your actions. When I was 14, a boy asked a friend of mine to attend a 21st birthday party with him. Her father said no when she asked him if she could go. He explained that they didn't know this boy's family or friends well and weren't sure she would be all right. Other friends invited to the party also had their parents say no for the same reasons. One of the parents arranged an alternative get-together for all the friends at their house on the same night to counter any disappointment.

- It's essential to control your own emotions. Just because your teen is angry and yelling doesn't mean you have to join in. Count to 10 and take deep breaths. If you can't deal with the situation at the time, make an excuse to leave and then discuss the incident when you've both calmed down.

- Spend time doing things together that everyone enjoys. While you're hiking, gardening, walking on the beach, visiting a museum, or having dinner out, you can have casual conversations. Establish what your teen is thinking and guide them. This is an excellent opportunity to make friends with your teen, as this will lay the groundwork for your future relationship with them when they are grown and gone.

- Eat dinner together around a table and leave your phones in another room, preferably on silent. Chatting together about your day and many other subjects will lay the foundation for discussing more complex things at other times.

- Keep an eye on your teen. If you see them behaving differently, avoiding friends and peers, or stopping doing things they usually enjoy, this may be a sign that all is not well. Approach them tactfully or find a time to ask them what is wrong. If they need professional help, feel free to get it for them.

APPRECIATING WHO TEENS ARE

Parents should remember to praise and thank their teens. Although they might scoff, they crave it as much as when they were younger. One simple but effective thing parents can do is list at least five items they appreciate about their teens every day. It can be something like when they get good grades, do an excellent job of mowing the lawn, tidy up without being asked, do someone a good turn, or something about their personality or appearance. You can do this privately, but what if you gave them a copy? They will feel encouraged. Imagine what it would be like if a significant person gave you a daily list of five things they love about you (Wilcox, 2021). This can also help to ease your relationship when things are strained.

As a parent, you should avoid looking at the negatives and being judgmental. Encourage every positive thing teens do. Don't be afraid of being vulnerable when you have moments of connection. That's a good time to tell your teen how much you value them.

DEVELOPING PROBLEM-SOLVING SKILLS IN TEENS

Teenagers must learn to deal with their problems to become responsible, mature adults. If parents continue to do this for them, they will never know how to resolve the challenges they may face in years to come. Some teens would instead find their solutions, even if this means making mistakes. Teens should be encouraged to stay calm and focus on practical solutions when dealing with problems.

Problem-solving will teach them to listen to others, consider others' opinions, become responsible and mature, and resolve conflicts. These are all essential life skills.

One way to encourage teens to develop problem-solving abilities is to stimulate their curiosity. Play games with them, challenge, and fight with them. Work constructively with them so they enjoy the process and grow.

Here are a few tips as to how parents can direct adolescents:

- Ask teens to identify the problem in their own words, immediately making it less overwhelming.

- Help them focus only on the situation, not their feelings or the person. This reduces anxiety and frustration, enabling them to face the problem head-on.
- Listen and allow them to express their wants, needs, and feelings about the situation.
- Encourage them to work out their own solutions and talk them through them. Some of their ideas might not be feasible, but getting them to work on solving the problem is essential.
- Discuss each solution to evaluate which ones work best. Encourage your teen to imagine possible outcomes of different scenarios so they can see how others would perceive them.
- Once your teen has selected a solution, please encourage them to implement it. Teens need to resolve problems independently to get used to finding solutions.
- Afterward, evaluate the outcome, considering some situations that might not resolve immediately. If things remain unresolved, then suggest your teen try some of their alternative solutions—this will develop tenacity.
- Then, discuss what worked well and what could be done in future similar situations. Praise your teen for their attempts, even if they didn't achieve their desired outcome. This will encourage them.

Influence of Technology on Problem-Solving

The technology could hinder problem-solving, especially when a practical, hands-on solution is required. A meme on social media captures this sentiment. There is a picture, probably taken in the 1970s, of a group of young men clustered around a car with the hood up. In the second photograph, two young men are sitting on a couch, phones in hand, watching television. The caption reads, "No wonder no one can fix their cars anymore."

Many of us have lost or never acquired essential life skills because we have relied excessively on technology. Plunged into a survival situation, most people wouldn't know what to do. Death or injury could result due to our lack of knowledge. Therefore, teaching teenagers practical, intellectual, and emotional skills is essential.

In the future, we are going to need practical skills. Parents must teach their teens to repair and fix things, grow vegetables, cook, sew, do plumbing or woodwork, look after children and animals, and more. Send them on courses if parents need help teaching them. This will not only develop their self-sufficiency, but it could also open them to possible job opportunities.

8

CASE STUDIES—SUCCESS STORIES

> *Holding on to anger is like grasping a hot coal with the intent of throwing it at someone else; you are the one who gets burned.*
>
> — BUDDHA

LIFE-CHANGING TEEN ANGER

In 11th grade, a teenage boy faced an angry outburst that reshaped his perspective. During lunch at the cafeteria, his meal was knocked over amidst a scuffle between some guys. They disregarded his pleas and trampled his belongings, fueling his rage. In the heat of the moment, he used his school bag to strike one of them. The aftermath was daunting: he was summoned to the principal's office, and despite his evident distress, the principal sternly reprimanded him. Exiting in a fury, he impulsively shattered a vase, resulting in his suspension.

The home was not a refuge that day. His parents, always his guiding lights, expressed their profound disappointment, making him feel even more isolated and misunderstood. A sharp comment from his mother pushed him to run away briefly, only amplifying his internal chaos.

Later, in the solitude of his room, an old video of his childhood became a mirror to his soul. Seeing his younger self, surrounded by the love and guidance of his parents, juxtaposed against the day's events, made him confront the vast gulf between who he was and who he had become. The stark realization prompted a heartfelt apology to his parents the following day. Their hesitant acceptance underscored the rift his actions had created.

Determined to mend things, he approached his school community with genuine repentance. The principal, while understanding, underscored that adolescence wasn't an excuse for unchecked emotions. She emphasized empathy, urging him to see things from the perspectives of his peers navigating similar emotional mazes. Heartened by her words, he sincerely apologized to his classmates. His earnest efforts led to the reconsideration of his suspension, and he emerged with a renewed understanding of the nuances of human emotions.

BUILDING A STRONGER TEEN-PARENT RELATIONSHIP

Seana had a close relationship with her daughter, but it looked like it would end when her daughter was in her mid-teens. The pair engaged in dreadful arguments interspersed with tense silences. Seana became worried about the future of their relationship. Seana decided she wouldn't let their relationship disintegrate and realized that, as the parent, it was up to her to make the first move.

She told her daughter she wanted to sit down with her and chat because things between them weren't great—and hadn't been for some time. Seana listed everything her daughter did to upset her and how it made her feel. When they sat down later that day, she could see that her daughter was on the defensive, so Seana calmly told her that she wanted to talk, not argue. They went through her list, discussing everything in detail. Seana's daughter then said she also had things she wanted to talk about. Seana was a little uncomfortable, but she listened to her daughter. They realized they needed to respect one another more and committed to that.

Seana realized that she needed to start treating her daughter like an adult. She had taught her daughter to respect herself and others, so she naturally wanted Seana to respect her, too. They didn't always get it right but learned to apologize, forgive, and move on.

Seana's daughter is now in her early 20s and in college. They once again enjoy a close relationship. She makes her mother proud and has many wonderful qualities. Seana says she's delighted she took the time to reassess her parenting style because it made all the difference.

BUILDING A RELATIONSHIP WITH A REBELLIOUS, TROUBLED TEEN

Marcia's stepdaughter was always a handful—and her father agreed. The stepdaughter was rebellious and disrespectful; they had to keep bailing her out. Marcia and her husband later divorced, and he moved away. However, Marica was concerned about her stepdaughter, as there were no other living relatives, and her stepdaughter's health was failing. She decided to keep in touch, offering what support she could.

Marcia soon realized that her stepdaughter's lifestyle wasn't to her liking—she drank, smoked, and possibly took drugs. Nevertheless, she tried to take an interest instead of verbally judging her. Over the years, Marcia discovered new qualities in her stepdaughter, praising her for her excellent attributes while overlooking the bad. After Marcia found out that her step-daughter played guitar, things improved.

Every day, Marcia listed five things—even small things—that she liked or was grateful for about her stepdaughter (Wilcox, 2021). For example, she put her plate into the sink after dinner, had pretty eyes, behaved herself in restaurants, and said thank you when Marcia did something for her.

Her stepdaughter moved out, but the two maintained contact. When her stepdaughter was raped, Marcia offered to help. Her stepdaughter declined but was grateful for Marcia's support. Marcia realized that her stepdaughter hadn't changed how she interacted with the rest of the world—she was still inclined to be wild and rebellious. But her stepdaughter did change how she related to Marcia. The two were still relatively close when her stepdaughter passed away.

Marcia discovered how little she knew her stepdaughter at the funeral. She met numerous people she hadn't realized were in her stepdaughter's life. She learned that her stepdaughter had been a loving, generous individual despite having a terminal illness. Marcia finally understood that the negative aspects of her stepdaughter's character had only manifested with Marcia and her husband. She realized their relationship with her might have been much better if they had interacted differently. They would also have experienced her kindness and compassion. When dealing with your offspring, your relationship with them is entirely up to you because you're the adult. It's not helpful to blame your child for difficulties in the relationship.

A FINAL REQUEST

With a better understanding of anger and how to manage it, you're well on the way to making the positive changes you want to see... and this is your chance to give that possibility to even more teens.

Simply by sharing your honest opinion of this book and a little about your own experience, you'll point new readers in the direction of the guidance they're looking for.

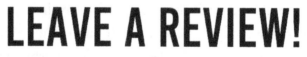

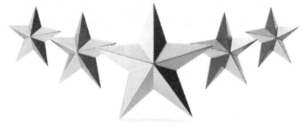

Thank you so much for your support. It makes a big difference.

Scan the QR code for a quick review!

CONCLUSION

 Let us not look back in anger, nor forward in fear, but around in awareness.

— JAMES THURBER

Anger is a strong emotion, but it's just that—a feeling, not a mental illness. Anger is one of the primary emotions but often manifests as hostility, aggression, explosive outbursts, and, in extreme cases, violence. It can harm people mentally, emotionally, and physically if uncontrolled. This is why anger gets so much attention. The intense feeling awakens the body's fight-or-flight response, ensuring our survival in life-threatening situations. The trouble is that this also releases stress hormones like cortisol and adrenaline that gear the body up for action. This is part of the reason why anger can be so destructive.

Teens get angry more frequently than adults. This is because adolescents' brains and central nervous systems are still developing. The limbic system, which lies deep in the brain and controls our emotions, matures faster than the prefrontal cortex, the seat of rational thought. This means that adolescents' emotions tend to override their logic. In addition, a structure in the limbic system called the amygdala signals the start of puberty by sparking the release of reproductive hormones. These are usually released in excess amounts, which increases teenagers' moodiness and sometimes unpredictable behavior. They get angry more quickly, feel misunderstood, and might perceive hostile intentions in the words and actions of others that have no basis in reality.

Today's teens live in a very stressful and challenging world. Adolescent anxiety and depression are rising steadily. The fallout from the COVID-19 pandemic, which affected this age group so badly that it even aged their brains prematurely, has increased their stress, especially if they lost caregivers.

Teens are under tremendous pressure to perform well academically and get into a good college. They need to cope with the physical changes their bodies are undergoing, navigate friendships and relationships that change continually as their characters form, decide on their careers, and cope with peer pressure, parent-teen conflict, sibling conflict, school shootings, and other forms of violence.

Adolescence is a tumultuous time filled with change, new opportunities, and adventures. Dopamine releases make teens seek out new and sometimes risky experiences. They want more freedom and responsibility but often need to make better choices due to their developing brains. This is all quite usual and natural as the brain prepares them to separate from their parents and become independent.

This is a lot for adolescents to take on, and it's no wonder many struggle to cope and show signs of stress, which may even become full-blown anxiety. It can lead to depression if not managed properly. Some teens try to self-medicate by turning to alcohol and drugs, which doesn't resolve the challenges and might worsen them. All this can fuel teen anger as they grow toward adulthood and try to find their place in the exciting but daunting adult world they will one day inhabit. Teens, especially boys, should not hesitate to ask for help if they need it.

There are plenty of things that parents and teenagers themselves can do to weather these exciting but often turbulent years. Teens need to understand and embrace their emotions and learn how to deal with triggers that make them angry. This might require therapy as some triggers are invisible, buried in the subconscious, and could relate to bad childhood experiences, abuse, bullying, etc.

Keeping an emotional journal enables teens to control their emotions and helps them understand the often negative thoughts underlying their behavior and angry outbursts. Getting enough sleep and exercise is very important, and it's a good idea to log off social media and electronic devices for a short period each day. Being creative, taking up a hobby, learning something new, or helping others are some of the ways teens can embrace the world and get a grip on their angry emotions and the actions they take as a result.

Anger can be managed with techniques such as deep breathing, three-step NPR action, tapping, controlled shaking, meditation, and relaxation exercises. Becoming mindful, developing self-awareness, and letting things go are all helpful.

Parents need to consider how their actions might inflame teenage anger. They should allow their teens to have greater autonomy while providing guidance and setting ground rules that can help protect their teens. It's best to use reasoning and discussions to enable teens to understand why their parents have established specific rules or boundaries.

Parents must set a good example for their teens so their children can emulate them. This includes things like managing emotions. Good communication is critical to establishing positive parent-child relationships that will endure into adulthood. Teens must be listened to, praised, encouraged, and given a solid foundation to build. They might not see the world as their parents do, but that's okay, too.

Many teens and parents have successfully negotiated their way through the teenage years with all their ups and downs, challenging experiences, and precious moments. While anger is a feature of these years, there is no reason why it should define parents, adolescents, or the future. I hope this book has helped you better understand your anger and diffuse it in the interest of better relationships.

REFERENCES

Abby, P. (2022). *I'm eighteen, and sometimes I want to scream at my older family members and get them to remember their adolescence.* [Comment on the video *The importance of having an unhappy adolescence*]. YouTube. https://www.youtube.com/watch?v=zcUI1Hk0GRU

Acosta, R. M. (2019, June 6). *I spent 7 years studying Dutch parenting—Here are 6 secrets to raising the happiest kids in the world.* CNBC. https://www.cnbc.com/2019/06/06/dutch-parenting-secrets-to-raising-the-happiest-kids-in-the-world.html.html

Acupuncture points—Pericardium 8. (n.d.). Acupuncture.com. http://www.acupuncture.com/education/points/pericardium/pc8.htm

Ambar. (2016). *There is a lot more that parents could, and should, be doing with their teens. As any parent with* [Comment on the blog post *What are some possible explanations for why teenagers might experience more anger and aggression than other age group? What are some tips for parents who are experiencing angry and aggressive teenagers?*]. Quora. https://www.quora.com/What-are-some-possible-explanations-for-why-teenagers-might-experience-more-anger-and-aggression-than-other-age-groups-What-are-some-tips-for-parents-who-are-dealing-with-angry-and-aggressive-teenagers?

Ambar. (2022). *Remember that our kids are our future. We need to be there for them* [Comment on the blog post *What are some possible explanations for why teenagers might experience more anger and aggression than other age groups?*]. Quora. https://www.quora.com/What-are-some-possible-explanations-for-why-teenagers-might-experience-more-anger-and-aggression-than-other-age-groups-What-are-some-tips-for-parents-who-are-dealing-with-angry-and-aggressive-teenagers?

American Academy of Pediatrics. (2021, December 21). *Mental health during COVID-19: Signs your teen may need more support.* HealthyChildren.org; American Academy of Pediatrics. https://www.healthychildren.org/English/health-issues/conditions/COVID-19/Pages/Signs-your-Teen-May-Need-More-Support.aspx

American Psychological Association. (n.d.). *Anger and aggression.* https://www.apa.org/topics/anger#:

Amritha K. (2021, July 5). *Anger foods 101: Foods that can cause anger, such as tomato, brinjal; and foods that help manage anger.* Bold Sky. https://www.bold sky.com/health/wellness/anger-foods-list-of-foods-that-can-cause-anger-and-foods-that-help-manage-anger/articlecontent-pf233333-137698.html

Anderson, M., & Jiang, J. (2018, May 31). *Teens, social media & technology 2018.* Pew Research Center. https://www.pewresearch.org/internet/2018/05/31/teens-social-media-technology-2018/

Anger issues in teen girls. (n.d.). Roots Renewal Ranch. https://rootsrenewal ranch.com/anger-issues-in-teens/#:

Anger myths. (n.d.). Counseling Services of Portland. https://www.counseling-portlandoregon.com/anger-issues/anger-myths/

Anonymous Contributor. (n.d.). *My teenage anger—Anger management story.* Www.breakthroughpsychologyprogram.com. http://www.breakthrough psychologyprogram.com/my-teenage-anger.html

Anxiety and stress in teens. (2021, April 12). Johns Hopkins All Children's Hospital. https://www.hopkinsallchildrens.org/ACH-News/General-News/Anxiety-and-Stress-in-Teens

Apter, P. (2009, January 19). *Teens and parents in conflict.* Psychology Today. https://www.psychologytoday.com/za/blog/domestic-intelligence/200901/teens-and-parents-in-conflict

Arabella. (2018). *The other day a random guy asked me 'when's the party?' I just looked at him because* [Comment on the video *Why are teens so moody?*]. YouTube. https://www.youtube.com/watch?v=du8siPJ1ZKo

Arain, M., Mathur, P., Rais, A., Nel, W., Sandhu, R., Haque, M., Johal, L., & Sharma, S. (2013). Maturation of the adolescent brain. *Neuropsychiatric disease and treatment, 9*(9), 449–461. https://doi.org/10.2147/ndt.s39776

AsapSCIENCE. (2016, February 14). *Why are teens so moody?* [Video]. YouTube. https://www.youtube.com/watch?v=du8siPJ1ZKo

Azab, M. (2018). *Why are teens so emotional?* Psychology Today. https://www.psychologytoday.com/us/blog/neuroscience-in-everyday-life/201810/why-are-teens-so-emotional

A Bag of Frogs and Eggshells With Anxiety. (2022) *I was having an awesome time with my friends and I was super excited to hang out because it was the* [Comment on the video *How to parent a teen from a teen's perspective*]. YouTube. https://www.youtube.com/watch?v=0vdPxLfAsqo

Basic emotions. (n.d.). Centre for Clinical Psychology Melbourne. https://ccp. net.au/basic-emotions/#:

Beresin, G. (2019, December 11). *11 self-care tips for teens and young adults.* MGH Clay Center for Young Healthy Minds. https://www.mghclaycenter. org/parenting-concerns/11-self-care-tips-for-teens-and-young-adults/

Beshoy. (2021). *It depends on what makes her angry. This advice is not just for you but for everyone. Rule no.1* [Comment on the blog post *How do I get my teenage daughter to stop being so mean when she is angry?*]. Quora. https:// www.quora.com/How-do-I-get-my-teenage-daughter-to-stop-being-so-mean-when-she-is-angry

Blakely, S. (2015, May 9). *Success story! Leadership solves angry teen problem!* LinkedIn. https://www.linkedin.com/pulse/success-story-leadership-solves-angry-teen-problem-steve-blakely

Bose, P. (2023, January 23). *Study finds high prevalence of depression and anxiety in children and adolescents during COVID-19 pandemic.* News-Medical.net. https://www.news-medical.net/news/20230123/Study-finds-high-preva lence-of-depression-and-anxiety-in-children-and-adolescents-during-COVID-19-pandemic.aspx

Brooks, L. (2017, April 25). *The differences between catecholamines and cortisol.* Sciencing. https://sciencing.com/differences-between-catecholamines-cortisol-7472976.html

Buckloh, L. M. (2018). *5 ways to know your feelings better (for teens).* Nemours TeensHealth. https://kidshealth.org/en/teens/emotional-awareness.html

Buddha quotes. (n.d.). BrainyQuote. https://www.brainyquote.com/quotes/ buddha_104025

Carlson, W., N., J., Rorabaugh, K., McCleaf, A., Mann, S., Osborne, J., Gardiner, K., & Thompson, M. (n.d.). *History of adolescence.* Sutori. https://www.sutori. com/en/story/history-of-adolescence--AzMPFnC6bYTyiBzPEcfzkfik

Chahar, P. (2021). *How can I overcome stress and anxiety?* Quora. https://www. quora.com/How-can-I-overcome-stress-and-anxiety

Charles, A., & Lamb, A. (2018, November 30). *Cary man sentenced to 12 years in prison on charges he killed his mother.* WRAL News. https://www.wral.com/ story/cary-man-sentenced-to-prison-on-charges-he-killed-his-mother-in-2015/18020758/

Charles Hurst Reinvention. (2022). *Suffering from chronic anger causes a few problems. First it impedes your progress.* [Comment on the video: *5 keys to controlling anger*]. YouTube. https://www.youtube.com/watch?v=KH3PHGjpo5Y

Chauncey, S. (2017, January 26). *Learning how to observe thoughts.* Living the Mess. https://www.livingthemess.com/learning-observe-thoughts/

Cherry, K. (2021, February 1). *Why toxic positivity can be so harmful.* Verywell Mind. https://www.verywellmind.com/what-is-toxic-positivity-5093958

Cherry, K. (2022, September 22). *What is mindfulness meditation?* Verywell Mind. https://www.verywellmind.com/mindfulness-meditation-88369

Chuck, E. (2023, April 27). *Two NC State students die of apparent suicide in 24 hours, bringing total number of suicides to 7 this school year.* NBC News. https://www.nbcnews.com/news/us-news/nc-state-student-dies-apparent-suicide-sixth-school-year-rcna81770

Cleveland Clinic. (2022, May 9). *Myelin sheath: What it is, purpose & function.* Cleveland Clinic. https://my.clevelandclinic.org/health/body/22974-myelin-sheath

Cody, T. (2022, January 28). *Wondering how to heal your emotional triggers? These 8 strategies will help.* iPECcoaching.com. https://www.ipeccoaching.com/blog/how-to-heal-emotional-triggers

Complex PTSD: Symptoms, behaviors, and recovery. (n.d.). MedicalNewsToday. https://www.medicalnewstoday.com/articles/322886#symptoms

Cooks-Campbell, A. (2020, July 15). *Triggers: Learn to recognize and deal with them.* BetterUp. https://www.betterup.com/blog/triggers

Cradlewise Staff. (2020, July 14). *How myelin sheath helps babies learn.* Cradlewise. https://cradlewise.com/blog/parenting/how-do-babies-learn-myelin-neurons-pregnancy-nutrition-tips

Cuncic, A. (2022, May 24). *"I hate myself": 8 Ways to combat self-hatred.* Verywell Mind. https://www.verywellmind.com/i-hate-myself-ways-to-combat-self-hatred-5094676

Cuncic, A. (2023, March 24). *How to be more present.* Verywell Mind. https://www.verywellmind.com/how-do-you-live-in-the-present-5204439

Dalai Lama Center for Peace and Education. (2014, May 13). *Daniel Siegel —The teenage brain* [Video]. YouTube. https://www.youtube.com/watch?v=TLULtUPyhog

Dangi, S. (2021). *Children are inherently curious in nature. When they go to school and* [Comment on the blog post *How do teenagers develop problem solving skills at the early stage of life?*]. Quora https://www.quora.com/How-do-teenagers-develop-problem-solving-skills-at-the-early-stage-of-life

DeFoore, W. G. (n.d.). *Teen anger management stories.* Anger Management Resource. https://www.angermanagementresource.com/teen-anger-management.html

Deschene, L. (n.d.). *To be beautiful means to be yourself. You don't need to be accepted by others. You need to accept yourself.* Tiny Buddha. https://tinybud dha.com/wisdom-quotes/to-be-beautiful-means-to-be-yourself-you-don-t-need-to-be-accepted-by-others-you-need-to-accept-yourself/

DeSilver, D. (2019, February 26). *The concerns and challenges of being a U.S. teen: What the data show.* Pew Research Center. https://www.pewresearch.org/fact-tank/2019/02/26/the-concerns-and-challenges-of-being-a-u-s-teen-what-the-data-show/

Dougherty, E. (n.d.). *Anger management.* Harvard Medicine. https://hms.harvard.edu/magazine/science-emotion/anger-management#:

Ducate, C. (2016). *We perpetuate a variety of outdated techniques that are no longer.* [Comment on the blog post *What are some possible explanations for why teenagers might experience more anger and aggression than other age groups?*]. Quora. https://www.quora.com/What-are-some-possible-explanations-for-why-teenagers-might-experience-more-anger-and-aggression-than-other-age-groups-What-are-some-tips-for-parents-who-are-dealing-with-angry-and-aggressive-teenagers?

Dunham, W. (2007, March 12). *Hormone paradox may help explain teen moodiness.* Reuters. https://www.reuters.com/article/us-puberty-hormone/hormone-paradox-may-help-explain-teen-moodiness-idUSN0940699220070312

DuPuis, C. (n.d.). *PC 8 acupuncture point theory.* Yin Yang House. https://yinyanghouse.com/theory/acupuncturepoints/pc8/#:

Edmunds, E. (2017, July 10). *The 4 components of mindfulness (SOAP)—Mindful therapy for anxiety.* Freedom from Anxiety. https://drellisedmunds.com/2017/07/10/1458/

Ehmke, R. (2016, May 16). *Tips for communicating with your teen.* Child Mind Institute. https://childmind.org/article/tips-communicating-with-teen/

Evans, L. (2020, January 21). *Emotions are messengers.* Elephant Journal. https://www.elephantjournal.com/2020/01/emotions-are-messengers/

Ferguson, C. (2015, July 20). *Why no-one can "make" you feel anything.* Mindset Trainer. https://carolineferguson.com/noone-can-make-you-feel-hurt/#:

Fight or flight response. (2021). Psychology Tools. https://www.psychologytools.com/resource/fight-or-flight-response/

Fisher, R. (2022, February 1). *Why teenagers aren't what they used to be.* BBC. https://www.bbc.com/future/article/20220124-why-teens-arent-what-they-used-to-be

Flannery, B. (2011, December 31). *Sources of conflict between parents and teenagers.* We Have Kids. https://wehavekids.com/parenting/Sources-of-Conflict-Between-Parents-and-Teenagers

Fleming, W. (2021, July 2). *Dear teen daughter, learn how to love yourself instead of being liked by others.* Parenting Teens & Tweens. https://parentingteensandtweens.com/teen-daughter-learn-to-love-yourself-not-be-liked/

Fries, L. (2022). *The importance of having the skills in problem solving is that the battery* [Comment on the blog post *What is the importance of having skills in problem solving?*]. Quora. https://www.quora.com/search?

Gary Zukav quotes. (n.d.). BrainyQuote. https://www.brainyquote.com/quotes/gary_zukav_637577

Gavin, M. (2019, February). *How much sleep do I need? (for teens).* Nemours TeensHealth. https://kidshealth.org/en/teens/how-much-sleep.html

Gerrie, H. (2020, June 10). *Our second brain: More than a gut feeling.* UBC Neuroscience. https://neuroscience.ubc.ca/our-second-brain-more-than-a-gut-feeling/

Gandhi, N. (2020, October 20). *Know your adversity quotient.* The Teenager Today. http://theteenagertoday.com/know-your-adversity-quotient/

Ghoul, K. T. (2017). *Our generation (gen z and some millennials) have the highest rates of suicide and depression and/or anxiety. Teens don't* [Comment on the video *Why are teens so moody?*]. YouTube. https://www.youtube.com/watch?v=du8siPJ1ZKo

Gladwin, S. (2020). *As a parent to a 17 year old, I think the real question being asked by parents of teenagers is* [Comment on the blog post *Why Do We Become More Angry with Our Parents in Teenage Years?*]. Quora. https://www.quora.com/Why-do-we-become-more-angry-with-our-parents-in-teenage-years

Golden, B. (2020, June 28). *Suppressed anger doesn't just go away.* Psychology Today. https://www.psychologytoday.com/za/blog/overcoming-destructive-anger/202006/suppressed-anger-doesn-t-just-go-away

Graf, S. (2020, November 17). *Roger Federer: The hothead discovers his zen.* TennisNet. https://www.tennisnet.com/en/news/roger-federer-the-hothead-discovers-his-zen

Gravitybread. (2014, August 7). *10 "grown up" sensory activities for an older child*

and/or teenager. Language During Mealtime. https://languageduringmeal
time.com/books-and-mealtime/10-grown-up-sensory-activities-for-an-
older-child-andor-teenager/

Gray, J. (2016, August 7). *How to fully release difficult emotions that hold you back.*
Jordan Gray Consulting. https://www.jordangrayconsulting.com/fully-
release-emotions-that-hold-you-back/

Guarnotta, E. (2021, December 14). *12 Signs of toxic parents & how to deal with
them.* Choosing Therapy. https://www.choosingtherapy.com/toxic-
parenting/

Hansen, R. (3011, September 26). *How to trick your brain for happiness.* Greater
Good. https://greatergood.berkeley.edu/article/item/
how_to_trick_your_brain_for_happiness

Herculano-Houzel, S. (2009). The human brain in numbers: A linearly scaled-
up primate brain. *Frontiers in human neuroscience, 3*(31). https://doi.org/10.
3389/neuro.09.031.2009

Hines, T. (2018, April). *Brain anatomy, anatomy of the human brain.* Mayfield
Brain & Spine. https://mayfieldclinic.com/pe-anatbrain.
htm#:~:text=Overview

How to cope with anger. (2023, June). Mind.org.uk. https://www.mind.org.uk/
information-support/types-of-mental-health-problems/anger/causes-of-
anger/

How to identify emotional triggers in 3 steps. (2021, May 15). Ridgeview
Behavioral Hospital. https://ridgeviewhospital.net/how-to-identify-
emotional-triggers-in-3-steps/

Hsieh, A. (2021). *Honestly? I think one of the reasons is partly because of ego, when
we think something looks easy enough, we* [Comment from the blog post *Why
do you get angry when playing video games?*]. Quora. https://www.quora.
com/search?q=%20living%20in%20their%20parent%E2%80%99s%20base
ment%20and%20finds%20more%20ways%20to%20annoy%20people&
type=answer

Hypothalamus: What it is, function, conditions & disorders. (2022, March 16).
Cleveland Clinic. https://my.clevelandclinic.org/health/articles/22566-
hypothalamus#:

Iyanla Vanzant quotes. (n.d.). BrainyQuote. https://www.brainyquote.com/
quotes/iyanla_vanzant_519947

Jakarian, N. (2020). *Dopamine is a neurotransmitter and a hormone. It is produced
by dopaminergic neurons in the brain from tyrosine from an* [Comment from

the blog post *What is the role of dopamine in the brain?*]. Quora. https://www.quora.com/What-is-the-role-of-dopamine-in-the-brain

Kasik, A. H. (2018, March 13). *11 expert tips to help put an end to self-judgments.* Brit + Co. https://www.brit.co/how-to-stop-self-judgments/

Kelley, E.T. (2017). *That's one of the biggest things a parent can do to help ease this period of transition. Parents need to* [Comment from the blog post *Why do we become more angry with our parents in teenage years?*]. Quora. https://www.quora.com/Why-do-we-become-more-angry-with-our-parents-in-teenage-years

Kernan, S. (2019). *Advice from one who graduated recently, don't get too invested or affected by your social standing as a teenager.* [Comment on the blog post *What's the worst part of being a teenager?*]. Quora. https://www.quora.com/Whats-the-worst-thing-about-being-a-teenager?no_redirect=1

Kevin, K (2017). *The school system needs to be changed. For me, even in elementary school, games made me learn more and I* [Comment on the video *Why are teens so moody?*]. YouTube. https://www.youtube.com/watch?v=du8siPJ1ZKo

Lawrence, E. (2022, October 25). *EFT tapping: What you need to know.* Forbes Health. https://www.forbes.com/health/mind/eft-tapping/

Leamey, T. (2022, April 5). *CDC survey finds the pandemic had a big impact on teens' mental health.* CNET. https://www.cnet.com/health/mental/cdc-survey-finds-the-pandemic-had-a-big-impact-on-teens-mental-health/

Li, P. (2023, January 30). *What is authoritative parenting? (Examples and comparisons).* Parenting for Brain. https://www.parentingforbrain.com/authoritative-parenting/

Liu, V., Rue, J., Fahmi, M., & Bent, D. (2018). *Points of you: Four friends from MIT on growing up.* Published By Authors.

Lowett, I. (2016). *At times, and now I'm willing to admit it, I became physically violent with my mother when she threatened to* [Comment on the blog post *Why do we become more angry with our parents in teenage years?*]. Quora. https://www.quora.com/Why-do-we-become-more-angry-with-our-parents-in-teenage-years

Lyness, D. (2015, July). *Peer pressure (for teens).* Nemours TeensHealth. https://kidshealth.org/en/teens/peer-pressure.html

Lyness, D. (2018). *How can I improve my self-esteem? (for teens).* Nemours TeensHealth. https://kidshealth.org/en/teens/self-esteem.html

Mariweem (2020). *And I've actually realized that, if you have love in yourself, it'll compel others to you. Just the simple act* [Comment on the video *The importance of an unhappy adolescence*]. YouTube. https://www.youtube.com/watch?v=zcUI1Hk0GRU

Marshall Goldsmith quotes. (n.d.). BrainyQuote. https://www.brainyquote.com/quotes/marshall_goldsmith_899333

Maydan, D. (2017). *We are constantly overthinking things. Does it really matter whether I picked up my shoes or remembered to put out* [Comment on the blog post *Why do we become more angry with our parents in teenage years?*]. Quora. https://www.quora.com/Why-do-we-become-more-angry-with-our-parents-in-teenage-years

McCarthy, C. (2019, November 20). *Anxiety in teens rising: What's going on?* HealthyChildren.org; American Academy of Pediatrics. https://www.healthychildren.org/English/health-issues/conditions/emotional-prob lems/Pages/Anxiety-Disorders.aspx

McKraken, P. (2020). *Start by granting the parent dignity and appreciation. Value for the many good things they do; emphasize* [Comment on the blog post *Why do we become more angry with our parents in teenage years?*]. Quora. https://www.quora.com/Why-do-we-become-more-angry-with-our-parents-in-teenage-years

Mehta, M. (2021, August 26). *Teenager anger management—What triggers it and how to help.* MichelleMehta.com. https://www.michellemehta.com/teenager-anger-management-what-triggers-it-and-how-to-help/

Mental Health America. (2019). *Helpful vs harmful: Ways to manage emotions.* https://www.mhanational.org/helpful-vs-harmful-ways-manage-emotions

Miller, L. (2017, September 11). *Is it anxiety or PTSD?* Liz Miller Counseling. https://lizmillercounseling.com/2017/09/anxiety-ptsd-difference/#:

Mindfulness Matters—Can living in the moment improve your health? (2017, June 28). NIH News in Health. https://newsinhealth.nih.gov/2012/01/mindful ness-matters

Mind Tools Content Team. (2022). *What are your values?* MindTools. https://www.mindtools.com/a5eygum/what-are-your-values

Moeller, H.-G. (2012). *Taoism.* Encyclopedia of Applied Ethics, 298–305. https://doi.org/10.1016/b978-0-12-373932-2.00217-9

Morin, A. (2022, September 20). *The top 10 social issues teens face in the digital world.* Verywell Family. https://www.verywellfamily.com/startling-facts-about-todays-teenagers-2608914

Morin, A. (2015, December 22). *7 myths about anger (and why they're wrong)*. Psychology Today. https://www.psychologytoday.com/za/blog/what-mentally-strong-people-dont-do/201512/7-myths-about-anger-and-why-theyre-wrong

Naseer, T. (2013, December 3). *A teenager's 4 lessons on how we can face any challenge*. Tanveer Naseer. https://tanveernaseer.com/4-lessons-on-how-we-can-overcome-any-challenge-alya-naseer/

Owens, E. (2020, October 12). *8 reasons why you should stop watching the news*. Antimaximalist. https://antimaximalist.com/stop-watching-the-news/

Padilla, J. (2022). *Suppressing anger takes a surprising amount of energy and effort, so this might mean missing out on* [Comment on the video *5 keys to controlling anger*]. YouTube. https://www.youtube.com/watch?v=KH3PHGjpo5Y

Paritosh, P. (2021). *As someone with social anxiety, I don't like going to places with large crowds, eating at fast food restaurants or* [Comment on blog post *What are the best ways to overcome stress and anxiety as a teenager?*]. Quora https://www.quora.com/What-are-the-best-ways-to-overcome-anxiety-and-stress-as-a-teenager

Peter. (2022). *I vividly remember the teenage years. My friends and I always acted as though we were intoxicated or weird* [Comment on the video *Why are teens so moody?*]. YouTube. https://www.youtube.com/watch?v=du8siPJ1ZKo

Plutchik's Wheel of Emotions: Exploring the Emotion Wheel. (2022, March 13). Six Seconds. https://www.6seconds.org/2022/03/13/plutchik-wheel-emotions/

Pratt, K. (2014). *Psychology tools: What is anger? A secondary emotion*. HealthyPsych. https://healthypsych.com/psychology-tools-what-is-anger-a-secondary-emotion/

Price-Mitchell, M. (2011, June 26). *What teens learn by overcoming challenges*. Psychology Today. https://www.psychologytoday.com/intl/blog/the-moment-youth/201106/what-teens-learn-overcoming-challenges

Rawhide Youth Services. (2015, September 18). *Teen anger and aggression —Causes and treatment*. https://www.rawhide.org/blog/wellness/teen-anger-aggression-causes-treatment/

RCC. (2016). *Teenagers think that they are old enough to make their own decisions. I, being a teenager myself, can vouch for* [Comment on the blog post *Why do we become more angry with our parents in teenage years?*]. Quora. https://www.quora.com/Why-do-we-become-more-angry-with-our-parents-in-teenage-years

Reynhamar, M. (2016). *Teenagers feel that parents are always out to get them, often correcting them, and telling them what to do and not* [Comment on the blog post *Why do we become more angry with our parents in teenage years?*]. Quora. https://www.quora.com/Why-do-we-become-more-angry-with-our-parents-in-teenage-years

Reynhamar, M. (2017). *For sure hormones play a part in teens lashing out, or other strong moods. But most of them are reachable with* [Comment on the blog post *Why do we become more angry with our parents in teenage years?*]. Quora. https://www.quora.com/Why-do-we-become-more-angry-with-our-parents-in-teenage-years

Rood, E. (2020, October 13). *Building emotional intelligence and self-awareness in teens.* Inspire Balance. https://inspirebalance.com/eq-self-awareness-teens/

Rowley, L. (2022, August 18). *Brainstorm summary.* Four Minute Books. https://fourminutebooks.com/brainstorm-summary/#:

Russell, J. (2019a, March 17). *Simple methods for emotional release.* Jazmine Russell. https://www.jazminerussell.com/blog/ways-to-release-pent-up-emotions

Safi'i, A., Muttaqin, I., Sukino, Hamzah, N., Chotimah, C., Junaris, I., & Rifa'i, Muh. K. (2021). The effect of the adversity quotient on student performance, student learning autonomy and student achievement in the COVID-19 pandemic era: evidence from Indonesia. *Heliyon, 7*(12), e08510. https://doi.org/10.1016/j.heliyon.2021.e08510

Sanyaolu, O. (2016). *For example, my parents try to force me to be religious, and they make me go to church with them.* [Comment on blog post: *Why do we become more angry with our parents in teenage years?*]. Quora. https://www.quora.com/Why-do-we-become-more-angry-with-our-parents-in-teenage-years

Sarah W. (2016, March 7). *How to love yourself.* Teen Line. https://teenlineonline.org/how-to-love-yourself/

Scheidies, C. (2017, April 18). *Common conflict situations for teenagers.* How to Adult. https://howtoadult.com/selfishness-teenagers-2746.html

Schmidt, M. (2014, September 6). *Connecting needs to feelings.* Maren Schmidt. https://marenschmidt.com/2014/09/connecting-needs-to-feelings/#:

Selva, J. (2018, March 8). *What is Albert Ellis' ABC model in CBT theory?* PositivePsychology.com. https://positivepsychology.com/albert-ellis-abc-model-rebt-cbt/#hero-single

Shameer, M. (2015, February 6). *10 useful tips to help your teens solve their problems.* Mom Junction. https://www.momjunction.com/articles/help-your-teen-solve-her-problems_00326769/

Sharon Salzberg quotes. (n.d.). BrainyQuote. *https://www.brainyquote.com/quotes/sharon_salzberg_527416*

Sherman, J. (n.d.). *Teen anxiety: Could it be nutrition related?* Jess Sherman. https://www.jesssherman.com/blog/teen-anxiety-is-it-nutritional

Siegel, D. (2017). Dr. Dan Siegel's Hand Model of the Brain. https://www.youtube.com/watch?v=f-m2YcdMdFw

Smith, K. (2022, October 21). *6 common triggers of teen stress.* Psycom. https://www.psycom.net/common-triggers-teen-stress

SoP. (2017, January 3). *Prefrontal Cortex.* The Science of Psychotherapy. https://www.thescienceofpsychotherapy.com/prefrontal-cortex/#:

Sparks, S. D. (2023, March 20). *One way to set students up for success: Let them sleep.* Education Week. https://www.edweek.org/leadership/one-way-to-set-students-up-for-success-let-them-sleep/2023/03#:~:text=While%20just%20over

Spector, N. (2019, November 6). *What is self-awareness? And how can you cultivate it?* NBC News. https://www.nbcnews.com/better/lifestyle/what-self-awareness-how-can-you-cultivate-it-ncna1067721

Stanborough, R. J. (2019, December 18). *Cognitive distortions: 10 examples of distorted thinking.* Healthline. https://www.healthline.com/health/cognitive-distortions#bottom-line

Stories of Eagle Village. (n.d.). *How a teen turned her life around: Becca's success story.* Eagle Village. https://eaglevillage.org/2018/01/19/beccas-success-story/

Swaminathan, N. (2007, March 12). Whatever!: Hormonal Reversal During Puberty Keeps Teens Totally Anxious. https://www.scientificamerican.com/article/hormone-reverses-in-puberty-causing-anxiety/#:

Talley, P.F. (2019). *It's the same way that I helped the little girl in group therapy (mentioned at the start of this post) overcame her fears.* [Comment on the blog post *How can I get rid of social anxiety and negativity?*]. Quora https://www.quora.com/How-can-I-get-rid-of-social-anxiety-and-negativity

TEDx Talks. (2020). *Be a better parent by partnering with your teen | David Kozlowski | TEDxSaltLakeCity* [Video]. YouTube. https://www.youtube.com/watch?v=uzhmBDrB8E4

Teenage peer pressure and 10 easy ways to say no. (2020, February 26). Elevations

RTC. https://www.elevationsrtc.com/b/feeditem/teenage-peer-pressure-and-10-ways-to-say-no/

Teen brains aged prematurely during COVID-19 pandemic. (n.d.). NIH COVID-19 Research. https://covid19.nih.gov/news-and-stories/teen-brains-aged-prematurely-during-covid-19-pandemic#:

Tengyuen, Ngan. "41 Quotes On Anger Management, Controlling Anger, And Relieving Stress." GeckoandFly. Last modified August 9, 2023. https://www.geckoandfly.com/27904/anger-management-stress-quotes/.

TheSpottedQuail. (2021). *Every time I go shopping, I get people stopping me to check my bags, who then say just checking you're shopping not stealing* [Comment on the video *Why are teens so moody?*]. YouTube. https://www.youtube.com/watch?v=du8siPJ1ZKo

Thought record sheet—7 column. (n.d.). McGill.ca. https://www.mcgill.ca/counselling/files/counselling/thought_record_sheet_0.pdf

Tiwari, A. (2023). *Living with a toxic parent is a nightmare and the fear you live with makes you extremely defensive. This defensive* [Comment on the video *Sadhguru left the girl speechless*]. YouTube. https://www.youtube.com/watch?v=BoHrwNrtGEk&t=309s

Tripple, M. (2023, May 10). *50 of the best parenting a teenager quotes.* Confessions of Parenting. https://confessionsofparenting.com/parenting-a-teenager-quotes/

Truschel, J. (2019, October 9). *8 foods that help with anxiety and stress.* Psycom. https://www.psycom.net/foods-that-help-with-anxiety-and-stress

Understanding anxiety in kids and teens. (2023, March 24). Mass General Brigham McLean Hospital. https://www.mcleanhospital.org/essential/anxiety-kids-teens

University of Rochester Medical Center. (2019). *Journaling for mental health.* Rochester.edu. https://www.urmc.rochester.edu/encyclopedia/content.aspx?ContentID=4552&ContentTypeID=1

University of Warwick. (2019, December 19). *Self awareness.* Warwick.ac.uk. https://warwick.ac.uk/services/wss/topics/selfawareness/

Welch, A. (2023, January 17). *A complete guide to meditation.* Everyday Health. https://www.everydayhealth.com/meditation/

When you're fighting with a friend... (2018, July 13). Kids Helpline. https://kidshelpline.com.au/teens/issues/fights-friends

Why shouldn't I avoid my negative emotions? (2021, February 11). Northstar-

Transitions.com. https://www.northstartransitions.com/post/why-shouldnt-i-avoid-my-negative-emotions

Wikipedia Contributors. (2019, January 4). *Adolescence*. Wikipedia. https://en.wikipedia.org/wiki/Adolescence

Wilcox, M. (2021). *I had a stepdaughter that was trouble with a capital T. She was rebellious, disrespectful and got into all sorts* [Comment on the blog post *I don't like my daughter. She is disrespectful and very negative. She clearly does not like me. How can I get her to be more positive and realize that I am not the enemy?*]. Quora. https://www.quora.com/I-don-t-like-my-daughter-She-is-disrespectful-and-very-negative-She-clearly-does-not-like-me-How-can-I-get-her-to-be-more-positive-and-realize-I-am-not-the-enemy

Wilderson, M. (n.d.). *How to deal with toxic parents*. Quora. https://www.quora.com/search?q=how%20to%20deal%20with%20toxic%20parents

Williams, M. (n.d.). *In encounters with your parents, just listen and ask for more information. Don't reply, don't argue* [Comment on the blog post *How can I know if my parents are toxic?*]. Quora https://www.quora.com/How-can-I-know-if-my-parents-are-toxic

Winterboer, C. (2017, October 31). *Starting young—The entrepreneurial success story of "Zesty Zandra."* Teen Entrepreneur. https://teenentrepreneur.co.za/starting-young-the-entrepreneurial-success-story-of-zesty-zandra/

Woodley, S. (2023, March). *Diffusing anger*.

Young, K. (2016, November 23). *Dealing with big feelings—Teaching kids how to self-regulate*. Hey Sigmund. https://www.heysigmund.com/how-to-self-regulate/

Your brain thrives on positivity. (2020, November 29). Sokya Health. https://www.sokyahealth.com/mood/your-brain-thrives-on-positivity/#rmation:

Zinn, J. K. (2019). *Mindfulness definition | What is mindfulness?* Greater Good. https://greatergood.berkeley.edu/topic/mindfulness/definition

IMAGE REFERENCES

Woodley, S. (2023). *Anger iceberg—Figure 1*.
Woodley, S. (2023). *Brain in general—Figure 2*.
Woodley, S. (2023). *PC 8 hand model—Figure 4*.
Woodley, S. (2023). *Teen brain—Figure 3*.

Made in the USA
Las Vegas, NV
26 November 2023

81604019R00098